Psychological Processes in Deaf Children with Complex Needs

Psychological Processes in Deaf Children with Complex Needs

An Evidence-Based Practical Guide

Lindsey Edwards and Susan Crocker

Jessica Kingsley Publishers
London and Philadelphia

First published in 2008
by Jessica Kingsley Publishers
116 Pentonville Road
London N1 9JB, UK
and
400 Market Street, Suite 400
Philadelphia, PA 19106, USA

www.jkp.com

Library of Congress Cataloging in Publication Data
Edwards, Lindsey, 1968-
    Psychological processes in deaf children with complex needs : an evidence-based practical guide / Lindsey Edwards and Susan Crocker.
        p. cm.
    Includes bibliographical references and index.
    ISBN 978-1-84310-414-8 (alk. paper)
    1. Deaf children--Psychology. 2. Deaf children--Family relationships. 3. Parents of deaf children. I. Crocker, Susan (Susan R.) II. Title.
    HV2391.E38 2008
    362.4'2019--dc22

                                                                    2007026012

British Library Cataloguing in Publication Data
A CIP catalogue record for this book is available from the British Library

ISBN 978 1 84310 414 8

Printed and bound in Great Britain by
Athenaeum Press, Gateshead, Tyne and Wear

For our daughters, Bethany, Hannah and Emilia,
without whom this book would have been
finished much sooner.

Acknowledgements

We would like to thank all the deaf children and families with whom we have worked over the last 12 years at the Nuffield Hearing and Speech Centre and Great Ormond Street Hospital for Children for helping us to advance our skills and knowledge about deafness and its application to clinical psychology. Without them this book would not have been possible.

We are also grateful to those people who made helpful comments and suggestions regarding the earlier drafts of this book: Roz Barker, Polly Carmichael, Ruth Merritt and Paul St John-Smith.

Contents

Foreword

'Well, it *is* complicated…'

A government programme officer once told me that parents of children with disabilities or special needs do not want to be told 'it's complicated'. In this volume, Lindsey Edwards and Susan Crocker point out that, although he was probably right, it does not mean that understanding and supporting such children is simple. When part of the equation is a significant hearing loss, which hinders communication and parent–child interactions, the situation can become very complicated indeed.

One of the challenges in raising and educating a deaf child is that a variety of 'experts' often operate on the basis of opinion, anecdote, and overgeneralizations. As a result, they fail to appreciate the extremely wide range of individual differences among such children, differences that far surpass those of hearing children. Understanding the needs and strengths of children who are deaf or hard of hearing is made even more complex by the fact that perhaps 40 per cent of them have physical, neurological or psychological issues either associated with, or frequently co-occurring with, hearing losses (and their etiologies). What we have been missing is a comprehensive description of the potential difficulties confronted by deaf children and their parents – and ways to go about avoiding and ameliorating them. Edwards and Crocker have now provided that description.

Deaf children often are viewed essentially as hearing children who cannot hear, with the implicit assumption that if communication barriers are removed development and education could proceed normally. As this volume ably points out, however, well…it's complicated. The importance of effective parent–child communication is perhaps the most central issue in understanding the development of deaf children, and it is front-and-centre as Edwards and Crocker review childhood psychological issues to which deaf children may be predisposed. Most refreshing is the way they clearly distinguish what we know and what we don't know. Parents of deaf and hard of hearing children frequently look to us for all the answers, but it is a rare professional who can bring parents to recognize that there often are no simple explanations for atypical behaviour, no method of communication that is ideal for all deaf children, and no school placement that always works.

Medical professionals are often unfamiliar with paediatric hearing loss, but also often suffer from a syndrome a biochemist I know described as 'they are not always right, but they are never uncertain'. Psychologists on the other hand, are often more likely to consider the whole child, examine family dynamics, and strive to put a child's hearing loss in a larger context. As researchers and clinicians, Edwards and Crocker are able to examine children's emotional, behavioural, and learning problems in terms of their functioning across domains.

This volume offers a broad perspective on psychological processes in children with complex needs. Armed with this valuable tool, professionals, parents and educators will be much better prepared to offer deaf and hard of hearing children the support and opportunities they deserve.

Marc Marschark
Center for Education Research Partnerships,
National Technical Institute for the Deaf,
Rochester Institute of Technology,
and School of Psychology,
University of Aberdeen

Preface

Since the mid-1990s when we both completed training as clinical psychologists, we have worked in services for deaf children. Indeed, for both of us, our first posts as qualified clinical psychologists were working with deaf children and young people referred to the service because of emotional, behavioural or learning problems. We were also both involved in the cochlear implant programme at the centre where we worked. At that time there were relatively few books or articles about the psychological aspects of deafness, and none that focused on the practical aspects of delivering a service to this group of children. Thus, we found ourselves in the challenging and unsettling position of having received no training on the specific needs of deaf children, and with few resources to guide us. Naturally we took every opportunity to attend seminars, workshops, conferences and so on, and established links with other psychologists working with deaf children around the UK for support and advice. However, we were often left feeling very unsure of whether our assessments and interventions were 'correct' and whether the service we were providing was the 'right' one. In the intervening years between then and now, the number of resources available to professionals working in the field of deafness has increased enormously. There are many thousands of research papers exploring the development of deaf children in terms of language, literacy, educational attainments, cognitive and neuropsychological functioning, socio-emotional development and so on. Equally there are now many books on these topics. Yet it seemed to us that there still remained a gap: there was no readily accessible source of information on how to go about assessing a deaf child experiencing psychological or learning difficulties, on how to work therapeutically with deaf children, or which strategies are the most suitable or effective in this group of children. So, after a number of years working in the field, we thought it was time we tried to fill that gap, with this book being the outcome.

Although we are both clinical psychologists whose profession would consider working with deaf children a highly specialized field, we are very aware that a wide range of other professionals work psychologically with deaf children, including counsellors, hearing therapists, educational psychologists and social workers. Teachers of the deaf and speech and language therapists are also frequently called upon to give advice or implement interventions for children with emotional or behavioural problems as part of their work with deaf children, input that could be considered psychological in nature. Therefore, our hope is that this book will be of interest and relevance to all those people who come into contact with deaf children and who provide a service of some kind for them.

At this point, it is necessary to make some comments regarding the title of this book, and its implications. As clinical psychologists, our training emphasized the 'scientist-practitioner' model, which stresses the importance of basing our clinical work on theoretical models of psychological functioning and good-quality research. More recently, the phrase 'evidence-based medicine (or practice)' has come into common usage, and is regarded by some as an ideal standard to which clinicians should aspire. Sackett *et al.* (1996, pp.71–72) define evidence-based medicine as 'the conscientious, explicit and judicious use of current best evidence in making decisions about the care of individual patients'. This definition has been expanded to 'the integration of best research evidence with clinical expertise and patient values' where patient values are the 'unique preferences, concerns and expectations each patient brings to a clinical encounter and which must be integrated into clinical decisions if they are to serve the patient' (Sackett *et al.* 2000, p.1). This requires the clinician to integrate knowledge gained from his or her own clinical experience and practice with the best available external clinical evidence from research. Research in this context can range from basic research, for example on the neuropsychological consequences of a syndrome causing deafness, to clinical research on the reliability and validity of a diagnostic test, to the efficacy and safety of therapeutic or preventative interventions. Research produces evidence, which similarly takes many forms. Evidence is anything that is used to determine or demonstrate the truth of an assertion and is typically used to support or refute a hypothesis. Evidence is also used in applied terms as guidance for a course of action. The National Institute for Clinical Excellence (NICE) produces guidelines on a range of treatments and interventions for medical conditions. It uses a recommendation grading scheme, A, B or C, with A being a recommendation based on the highest level of clinical evidence. It also classifies some recommendations as 'good practice points', which are based on the clinical experience of the group of experts who contributed to the guidelines. The NICE grading scheme is based on the scheme formulated by the Outcomes Group of the NHS Executive (1996). From our perspective it is helpful to consider the evidence from studies involving deaf children within this framework, so it is summarized here for reference:

- *Grade A*: At least one randomized controlled trial as part of a body of literature of overall good quality and consistency addressing the specific recommendation without extrapolation.

- *Grade B*: Well-conducted clinical studies (including well-designed controlled studies without randomization, quasi-experimental studies, correlational and comparative studies) but no randomized clinical trials on the topic of recommendation; or extrapolated from a randomized controlled trial or meta-analysis of randomized controlled trials.

- *Grade C*: Expert committee reports or opinions and/or clinical experiences of respected authorities. This grading indicates that directly applicable clinical studies of good quality are absent or not readily available.

In this type of scheme, evidence from randomized controlled trials (where patients are randomly assigned to the intervention or some form of comparator group), or systematic reviews where there is homogeneity of studies, are considered the gold standard for both diagnosis and intervention. Where neither the patient nor the person providing the intervention knows who is in which group, the study is also considered 'double-blind', conferring an even greater level of respectability in terms of quality of evidence. When we consider the evidence available for deaf children, we shall see throughout the book that this gold standard has yet to be met. However, there are a number of very good, valid reasons for this. First, deafness is a relatively rare condition, so the numbers of participants available for research of this nature are limited. Second, the population of deaf children is highly heterogeneous in terms of the aetiology of deafness, degree of hearing loss, the language used by the child, the presence of additional disabilities and the type of schooling received, to name but a few. These all have an impact on the child's development, and would need to be accounted for in any appraisal of the impact of an intervention. We need to be mindful of the fact that variations in social, emotional and cognitive development among deaf children are greater than the differences between these children and the hearing population. If we narrow things down further, and wish to investigate the efficacy of an intervention for deaf children with a specific disorder, for example attention deficit hyperactivity disorder (ADHD), we then have to consider whether our diagnostic criteria will produce a homogeneous study population. This is unlikely when the causes of such disorders are complex, multi-factorial and based on multi-dimensional, behaviourally defined criteria. Third, there are a number of ethical and practical reasons why randomized controlled trials are problematic. For example, thinking about cochlear implantation in children, it is hard to imagine any parent who is told that their child is likely to benefit from a cochlear implant, agreeing to be randomly assigned to a no-treatment or waiting-list control group, in the interests or furthering scientific knowledge. Equally it is impossible to prevent therapists, parents and even the children themselves from being aware of what type of intervention the children are receiving, so prevention or intervention studies cannot be double-blinded. Some would argue that studies of this type fail to answer the research questions and potentially do the study population a disservice, as they discourage the clinician from developing individualized formulations and intervention strategies based on the specific problems, life circumstances and desires of the individual.

Throughout this book, we have presented research evidence, of whatever type is available, that is of relevance to clinical practice when working with deaf children with psychological problems. On the whole, research in this area involves cohort or case series studies (where a group of children are followed over a period of time to monitor progress), cross-sectional studies (for example where deaf children are compared with hearing children on specific indices), or case reports (where a single, highly unusual case is described in detail). Although not meeting the 'gold standard', at the present time, this is the reality of the state of evidence available to us. However, there is much to be said in favour of the evidence base that has accumulated, as it provides us with many ideas for 'good practice points', and it is these that we have highlighted throughout the following chapters. We also acknowledge that some of the suggestions for assessment or intervention are based on our own clinical experience of working with deaf children, and are personal views. Hume [1748] (1999) said, 'A wise man...proportions his belief to the evidence.' Our aim is that in time, research will provide us with evidence to guide our clinical work to an increasing extent.

Having presented our thoughts on evidence-based practice, we now also need to clarify our position in relation to the diagnosis of mental health and other disorders amongst deaf children. Controversy continues to exist regarding the appropriateness, utility and even ethicality of diagnosing mental health disorders, with some strong opposition amongst psychologists and other professionals. Throughout this book we have tried to strike a reasonable balance between the medical and cultural models of deafness. In brief, the former model views deafness as a disability to be ameliorated if possible, whereas in the latter, deafness is viewed as a positive state, not to be changed. It has become standard practice to distinguish between 'deaf' as a descriptive, audiological term, and 'Deaf', with a capital D, to denote membership of the Deaf community and we have also used this convention. Whilst we would not wish to impose the medical model on any deaf child or family for whom this was not wanted, the reality of our experience of working with deaf children is that some experience significant additional medical, physical and psychological difficulties, which bring them into frequent contact with health services, including psychology services. Parents of children with emotional, behavioural or learning difficulties often seek a diagnosis or label for their child's problems, as this is likely to give them access to the additional specialist educational and social services they need. It can also give validity to their concerns, and a way of communicating their child's difficulties, in a manner that is more readily understood and accepted by others. Therefore, some of the chapters in this book do present a 'medical' perspective on psychological problems, and in particular how they can be diagnosed in deaf children.

In this context, it is helpful to understand the way in which common mental health and developmental disorders are usually diagnosed. The *Diagnostic and Statistical Manual of Mental Disorders* (*DSM*) is a handbook for mental health professionals that lists different categories of mental disorder and the criteria for diagnosing them, according to the publishing organization, the American Psychiatric Association (APA). The *DSM* has gone through five revisions since it was first published in 1952. The last major revision was the *DSM-IV* published in 1994, although a 'text revision' was produced in 2000. The *DSM-V* is due for publication in approximately 2011. The mental disorders section of the *International Statistical Classification of Diseases and Related Health Problems* (*ICD*) is another commonly used guide, and the two classifications use the same diagnostic codes. The *ICD* is published by the World Health Organization (WHO). Since the 1990s, the APA and WHO have worked to bring the *DSM* and the relevant sections of *ICD* into concordance, but some differences remain. The *ICD* is revised periodically and is currently in its tenth edition. The *ICD-10*, as it is therefore known, was developed in 1992 to track mortality statistics. *ICD-11* is planned for 2014. Annual minor updates and three-yearly major updates are published by the WHO. The *ICD* is part of a 'family' of guides that can be used to complement each other, including also the *International Classification of Functioning, Disability and Health*, which focuses on the domains of functioning (disability) associated with health conditions, from both medical and social perspectives. In the UK, the *ICD* system is customarily used. Where relevant, we have used the diagnostic criteria from these classifications to guide good practice in the assessment and diagnosis of mental health and developmental disorders in deaf children.

However, whilst diagnostic manuals of this sort provide us with guidelines and criteria by which diagnoses should be made, they do not give any indication of the best tools to use to compare the 'symptoms' of a particular child with the criteria for a specific diagnosis. In other words, it is left to the clinician to decide which psychometric test, questionnaire or other assessment method is most likely to identify the disorder correctly. In some medical fields 'gold standards' for diagnostic tests with high positive predictive value (where the chances of a disease or disorder being present are high given a positive test result) are being established. Where presenting problems are behavioural or psychological in nature, this is much more challenging. In the field of childhood deafness where there is little guidance, there is a great need for research to establish the validity and reliability of assessment tools intended for the hearing population when used with deaf children.

Through this book we hope we will convey our enthusiasm for working with deaf children and their families, in what is a challenging, stimulating and rewarding field. Knowledge and understanding of the psychological consequences of childhood deafness is increasing rapidly but there is a great need for further good research on the best ways to help deaf children experiencing psychological problems. New evidence, as it accumulates, is likely to have implications for our clinical practice and we look forward to reflecting on this volume in a few years' time, saying how differently and how much better we can do things now. This is the way of the future.

Lindsey Edwards and Susan Crocker

Note on terminology

The terms deaf/ness and hearing-impaired/impairment are used interchangeably throughout this book and refer to the full range of degree of hearing loss from mild to profound. When describing research we have tended to use the terms used by the authors, and the term 'hard of hearing' is used as defined in specific contexts.

1 The Experience of Childhood Deafness

In this chapter we aim to provide a broad outline of the field of deafness including the main types and causes of deafness, methods for diagnosing hearing loss and the most common treatments for permanent hearing loss. We will briefly introduce a number of common technical terms that will be used throughout the remainder of the book. The remainder of the chapter will consider the impact of a diagnosis of permanent hearing-impairment on a child and his or her family in some depth, as this underpins so much of the involvement of clinical psychologists with deaf children. Some of the topics covered are of such significance to the development of deaf children, and their future psychological well-being that the issues are considered further in separate chapters later in the book. The aim of the following sections is to given an indication of the diverse and far-reaching consequences of childhood deafness, on the children themselves, their parents and brothers and sisters.

Finally, the role that psychologists may be asked to play in the lives of these children and families, and the ways in which working therapeutically with them may differ from other children, will be discussed.

The epidemiology, types and causes of childhood deafness
Prevalence

Fortnum and Davis (1997) have estimated that in the UK, 1.12 babies in every 1000 live births have a congenital, permanent hearing loss of 40dB (decibels) or greater across the frequencies 0.5, 1, 2 and 4kHz (kilohertz). This increases to 1.33 per 1000 children by the age of five years. Around 21 per cent of these children have a profound hearing loss from birth. In order to hear speech sounds, children need to be able to hear sounds of approximately 30–60dB across the frequencies 250–8000Hz (this is an over-simplification but gives an idea of the situation). Therefore, in an average primary school of around 400 pupils, you might expect one child every two to three years to have a hearing loss, which (if left unaided) would impact their language development and therefore limit full access to the normal curriculum.

Types of deafness

There are two main types of deafness. The first is conductive hearing loss, where there is a problem with sound being transmitted through the outer ear (comprising the pinna and ear canal) and/or the middle ear (the tympanic membrane – eardrum and a 'box' in the bone of the skull containing three tiny bones or 'ossicles', the malleus, incus and stapes). The most common reason for a conductive loss in children is the condition 'glue ear', or otitis media with effusion, where the middle ear fills with fluid, preventing the ossicles from vibrating and transmitting the sound waves. Glue ear typically results in fluctuations in hearing levels, of up to around 50dB hearing loss, so can have a significant impact on a child's perception of spoken language. There are a number of other causes of conductive hearing loss, but these are much rarer.

The second type of hearing loss is called sensori-neural deafness. It is caused by malfunctioning of the cochlea (the inner ear) and/or the nerve that transmits the sound signal from the cochlea to the auditory and other higher centres of the brain. Most sensori-neural deafness is a result of damage to the cochlea and is permanent. In a proportion of children with this type of hearing loss, hearing levels gradually deteriorate over time, producing a progressive hearing loss.

Causes of sensori-neural deafness

The great majority (possibly around 75%; Graham 2004) of cases of congenital sensori-neural deafness are caused by genetic abnormalities, either dominant or recessive. Some genetically caused conditions have deafness as the only or primary abnormality, whereas in approximately 30 per cent of cases the deafness is part of a wider constellation of physical abnormalities, making a syndrome. The most common syndromes resulting in significant sensori-neural hearing loss include Waardenburg syndrome, Usher syndrome, Pendred's syndrome and CHARGE association.

Other causes of congenital hearing loss arise from infection such as cytomegalovirus (CMV), toxoplasma virus and syphilis infection whilst the foetus is developing. Prematurity is also a significant cause of sensori-neural deafness and is also often associated with other physical abnormalities, medical problems and learning difficulties.

Another relatively frequent cause of deafness during childhood is meningitis. Often the only apparent consequence of the illness is the hearing loss, but a complete spectrum of disability can arise from it, from dual sensory loss, to septicaemia resulting in the need to amputate limbs, to significant learning disabilities.

Diagnosing sensori-neural hearing loss

When we have seen a family with one or more deaf children who were being referred for psychological intervention, one of the experiences that has often had a lasting impact has been the time when they were told their child is deaf. Parents frequently recall the period during which the diagnostic tests were being carried out as being highly stressful and distressing. The moment when a permanent hearing-impairment is confirmed by a doctor or audiologist can be experienced as devastating. Therefore, when working with families it is important to have a basic knowledge of the tests their child may have undergone, and is likely to have to undergo again at various times in the future.

Behavioural tests

The ages given are approximate and depend on the developmental level of the child:

1. *Behavioural Observation Audiometry (BOA)* for children up to around seven months, or older if they cannot give an intentional response to sound. Behaviours observed include startling to loud sounds or stirring from sleep.

2. *Visual Response/Reinforcement Audiometry (VRA)* for children between seven months and around three years. The child responds to sounds by turning his or her head towards a loudspeaker to their left or right, and are rewarded by a visual display, for example twinkling lights, or a moving toy on top of the speaker.

3. *Play Audiometry* for children from two to three years upwards. When a sound is heard the child carries out an action such as putting a marble in a marble race, or a man in a wooden boat, or some other 'game'.

Electrophysiological tests

1. *Oto-Acoustic Emissions (OAEs) (cochlear echoes)* assess the function of the hair cells in the cochlea.

2. *Auditory Brainstem-evoked Response Audiometry (ABR)* assesses information on the electrical activity generated along the nerve pathway (the brainstem) to the brain using electrodes placed on the scalp. The test is performed whilst the infant is asleep, or requires sedation/anaesthesia in older children.

3. *Electrocochleograpy (EcoG)* needs to be performed in hospital under general anaesthetic, and measures the tiny electrical signals generated in the cochlea and at the start of the hearing nerve.

4. *Tympanometry* assesses middle ear function and provides information regarding conductive hearing loss.

Interventions for hearing loss

Not surprisingly, there are different interventions that are appropriate for different types of hearing loss. The most common ones are outlined below.

Conductive hearing loss

Glue ear, or otitis media with effusion, affects one in four children at some point from infancy to around 10 or 11 years of age. If it becomes a persistent, recurrent problem it may become necessary to remove fluid from the middle ear by surgical means – insertion of 'grommets' or ventilation tubes in the affected ear(s). After a period of months, in almost all cases, the grommet is extruded naturally. In many children, surgery needs to be repeated, sometimes several times, until the child has 'grown out' of the problem.

Sensori-neural hearing loss
CONVENTIONAL HEARING AIDS (HAs)

Hearing aids, both analogue and digital, work by amplifying environmental sounds, including speech sounds. Though louder, sounds may not be clearer, especially if the 'target' sounds are heard in the context of background noise. Digital aids, with their newer, more sophisticated technology can be programmed to meet the specific needs of the child, and although they often provide better access to speech than analogue aids, are still not sufficient in a significant proportion of children.

COCHLEAR IMPLANTS (CIs)

Unlike analogue or digital hearing aids, cochlear implants do not amplify sound. Instead the implant directly stimulates the auditory nerve using electrical signals. A series of tiny electrodes are surgically inserted into the cochlea, connected to a 'receiver' package that sits under the scalp behind the ear. The external parts of the system comprise a *microphone*, which picks up sounds, a *speech processor*, which processes the sounds, changing them into electrical signals that pass along a lead to the *coil*, which transmits the signal to the receiver package. By adjusting the settings of the receiver package the tiny current that stimulates the auditory nerve is set or 'tuned' to meet the specific auditory needs of the child, producing a sensation of sound.

Clinical psychologists are increasingly involved, along with a wide range of other professionals, in cochlear implant services in the UK, providing a clinical service to children undergoing assessment for the procedure, those who receive an implant and their families. Psychology also has an important role to play in research in this field, therefore a whole chapter (Chapter 6) is devoted to the topic.

BONE-ANCHORED HEARING AIDS (BAHAs)

Conventional hearing aids conduct sound through the ear canal and the middle ear. In contrast, a BAHA conducts sound through the skull bone, of which the cochlea is part. This allows sound to be transmitted more directly to the inner ear, in children for whom conventional HAs are not suitable, perhaps because of the anatomy of the outer and/or middle ear. The BAHA sound processor clips on to an 'abutment' attached to a small titanium screw that has been implanted in the skull just behind the ear.

The impact of deafness on the child and family

Diagnosis, adjustment and coping

The diagnosis of a permanent hearing loss is of major significance to families of both deaf and hearing parents. Parents can typically recall exactly where, when, how and by whom they were given the diagnosis many years after the event. With the national roll-out of the Universal Newborn Hearing Screening Programme in the UK, which was completed by mid-2005, the age at which sensori-neural hearing losses are identified is becoming much lower than previously, when it was not uncommon for parents to experience difficulty obtaining a reliable diagnosis before their child had entered the education system. When parents feel they have had to fight for a diagnosis, finally receiving it may bring a sense of relief. However, a mixture of emotions is common, typically being negative and very strong. In a review of the research literature on the social and emotional consequences of Universal Newborn Hearing Screening, Yoshinaga-Itano (2001) considers both the positive and negative implications of early diagnosis. She concludes that overall, parents do not experience greater levels of clinical stress as a result of screening than new parents do generally, especially when appropriate and timely intervention is provided.

A balance is needed between acknowledging the enormity of the impact of the diagnosis and not presenting it as an insurmountable problem. Parents may need help to empower themselves and avoid a perception of helplessness; the reactions and responses of parents (and the wider family) to deafness can cause as much of a problem as the deafness itself. Whilst early diagnosis can be very positive in terms of mobilizing services and maximizing auditory input (and therefore speech and language outcomes), some parents may feel that this knowledge of their child's disability prevents them from bonding with their baby. Indeed, despite the empirical research evidence suggesting the opposite, anecdotal evidence from the National Deaf Children's Society (NDCS) internet discussion forum ('Parent Place') indicates high levels of distress and anger amongst some mothers whose child was diagnosed with a hearing loss within a few days or weeks of birth (see www.ndcs.org.uk/applications/discussion). Wanting time to bond with their baby before being thrown into the turmoil that the diagnosis of deafness engendered, was a common theme. Careful exploration of these issues is often needed when taking a history and working therapeutically with families where a deaf child is presenting with emotional or behavioural difficulties. Unresolved feelings around having a deaf child, and the timing of diagnosis, can have a significant impact on the functioning and well-being of the child, along with influencing family dynamics.

Whilst the diagnosis of deafness may be perceived negatively by many parents, this should not be assumed. In particular, where one or both parents are themselves deaf, the diagnosis may be welcomed, but again this is not always the case and therefore should not be assumed. For hearing parents, if the deafness has a genetic aetiology, the birth of subsequent children may be very stressful. Parents may want the baby's hearing tested as soon as possible, or may wish to wait until they have had time to bond with their baby. Either way, most parents will have learnt many skills in terms of parenting a deaf child and negotiating the relevant health care and educational services, which may make bringing up a second deaf child less daunting.

EMOTIONAL RESPONSES TO DIAGNOSIS – PARENTS

Some authors have likened the process of coming to terms with the diagnosis of deafness to that of adjustment to bereavement, with a series of stages: shock, denial, grief, anger, guilt and finally resolution (e.g. Webster 1994). However,

Kurtzer-White and Luterman (2003) caution against this due to fundamental differences in the nature of grief following death compared with ongoing parental grief. Many parents do not appear to follow this orderly pattern of stages, or anything resembling it. This should not be considered 'abnormal' or dysfunctional, but rather a normal variant of individuals' responses to stress and their coping styles. In whatever way one theoretically conceptualizes the emotional responses of parents to the diagnosis, some parents do present with prolonged difficulty adjusting to the diagnosis. Currently there is a paucity of research on the long-term effects of chronic grief and its impact on parent–child bonding, especially in the context of permanent hearing loss. The exception is a pilot study by Pipp-Siegel (2000) who found a trend towards a significant difference between the ages at which hearing loss was identified for those parents who had resolved their grieving and those who had not; earlier identification was associated with faster grief resolution. Pipp-Siegel suggests that the resolution of grief may be strongly related to the language development of the child and improvements in maternal bonding. Pipp-Siegel also strongly advocates the involvement of professionals with appropriate counselling skills and knowledge of deafness, to help families cope with the diagnosis and its implications.

Therapeutically, the psychologist can usefully explore the coping strategies parents have used in the past to deal with difficult situations, and consider how they may be helpful now. Where parents (and other close relatives) do react with strong feelings of anger or helplessness, the situation is sometimes compounded by the amount of new information and skills to be taken on board, for example the results of audiological assessments and how to use hearing aids. Other emotions expressed by families may include fear, anxiety, confusion or even foolishness, all of which may have long-term consequences for the psychological well-being of the child and family.

Beazley and Moore (1995) argue that parents' reactions are very unpredictable, and may actually be the result of the way in which the professionals involved have interacted with them. These authors warn that parents who appear to be coping well may be accused of or seen as being in denial. If parents do display grief, misery or depression, professionals may believe that to be the normal response and therefore assume there is no need to offer help or support. Finally, Beazley and Moore suggest that 'bereavement' theories of adjustment allow professionals to abrogate responsibility – in other words, the parents' expressions of anger or depression may be interpreted as due to the diagnosis of deafness, rather than due to the way in which they were told of the diagnosis or the difficulties achieving an accurate diagnosis.

When working psychologically with families, it is important to be sensitive to these issues and be aware of the impact of the diagnosis itself in addition to the parents' experience of the health care system and the wider system of professionals.

EMOTIONAL RESPONSES TO DIAGNOSIS – CHILDREN

In considering the emotional response to the diagnosis of permanent deafness, it is important to bear in mind the child's reaction to his or her own deafness. By no means all deafness is congenital and the diagnosis made whilst the child is in his or her infancy and unlikely to recollect the experience. When deafness is caused suddenly, most commonly as the result of meningitis, or is, for example, as a result of widened vestibular aqueduct syndrome, the child may experience very strong emotions. Children may show signs of anxiety, fear, anger or depression, or show behavioural disturbance. They may become withdrawn and suffer poor self-esteem as their communication and language skills deteriorate, and their self-confidence is knocked. In these circumstances the psychologist can play an important role in supporting the child and his or her family, offering therapeutic intervention when the emotional responses are severe and mental health problems ensue. Input needs to take into account the child's developmental age (which may differ markedly from their chronological age) and stage in childhood, for example major transition points such as starting or changing school.

Attachment

The concept of attachment, developed by John Bowlby in animals and researched in human infants by Mary Ainsworth, has been explored in the context of deaf children by a small number of researchers. In the 'strange situation' paradigm (Ainsworth and Bell 1970), the infant is exposed to a series of entrances and exits from the room by his or her mother and an unfamiliar adult, and the child's reactions to these separations and reunions are observed. On the basis of these reactions the child's attachment to his or her mother is classified as secure, avoidant, ambivalent or disorganized. Although not always explicitly stated, the basic tenet of research on attachment in deaf infants has been the assumption that deafness must somehow (negatively) influence the development of attachment between the deaf infant and his or her mother. In an early dissertation, Greenberg (1978) examined the influence of method of communication (oral versus total) and communicative competence on the attachment relationship between profoundly deaf infants and their hearing mothers. He found patterns of attachment similar to those reported for hearing children, but also reported significant relationships between communication method (not competence) and the quality of interactions, maternal stress and the child's level of social skills. In another dissertation, Spangler (1987) used the Ainsworth 'strange situation' paradigm and found a higher incidence of avoidant and resistant classifications between the deaf children and hearing mother dyads compared with hearing dyads. The non-secure attachments were associated with less resolved grief in the mothers and poorer coping but there was no relationship between the quality of attachment and the type of communication used with the child.

More recently, Pressman *et al.* (2000) reported a longitudinal study of 21 hearing-impaired toddlers and 21 hearing controls, which employed a questionnaire measure of emotional availability (bonding) between mother and child, focusing on maternal sensitivity and warmth, maternal structuring of the child's behaviour/intrusiveness and maternal frustration or hostility. They reported no differences in emotional availability of the mothers in the two groups, but interestingly, in both groups higher maternal sensitivity predicted faster language gains. Hadadian (1995) used an observational rating of the security of attachment and found a negative correlation between security of attachment and parental attitudes towards deafness.

Thus, from the sparse literature available, it appears that attachment patterns in young deaf children may be distinguishable from those of their hearing peers, and that the quality of the relationship between the child and his or her mother may have implications for the child's development of communication and language skills.

From a clinical perspective, we have only very occasionally seen cases where there is an obvious, severe disturbance of the attachment relationship between a hearing mother and deaf child. In these cases, there have usually been clear indications of unresolved grief. However, frequently the deafness has been only one of a number of other severe disabilities, and therefore the impact of the deafness per se has been hard to gauge. In working therapeutically with deaf children where the attachment relationship appears to be a contributory factor to the child's difficulties, intervention should focus on improving the parent's sensitivity to their child's communicative attempts. 'Scaffolding' of the child's language is a useful strategy whereby the adult copies the child's attempt at communication, then extends it very slightly, by using one or two additional words (or signs), and waiting for the child to respond or communicate something else. The adult's behaviour needs to be rhythmic, timely, flexible and adaptable to the demands and needs of the child, following the child's lead rather than being directive and intrusive. The use of eye contact, facial expression and physical contact in play are essential, but appropriate setting of boundaries and containment of frustration are equally important.

ommunication and language

Language and communication are by no means synonymous. Children can develop some communication skills in the absence of language skills. For example, body language, gestures and facial expression can all convey considerable information – about what the person wants, what they are feeling and so on. Clearly, though, in order for communication skills to develop to the most sophisticated, complex level associated with human beings, language skills must also be acquired to the highest level possible for that individual.

COMMUNICATION

Communication skills develop from the earliest days of life. Babies spend a lot of time looking at faces, particularly their mother's, whilst being held in her arms. Babies respond to changes in facial expression, quickly learning to copy them and to take turns in the 'conversation' with their parents. This moves on to conversations using sounds such as cooing and gurgling, then 'baby talk', using a higher pitch, slower tempo and more lyrical rhythm than normal speech. A significant proportion of parents of deaf babies describe feeling unsure or deskilled when communicating with their baby or young child. Deaf babies typically follow normal patterns of pre-verbal communication, including copying facial expression, gestures, babbling and joint attention, thus sometimes leading parents to doubt the diagnosis of hearing impairment. Alternatively, knowing their child is deaf may cause parents to believe there is no point copying their babbling, using baby talk or later on using normal spoken language. However, deaf and hearing-impaired babies can and do respond to normal pre-verbal communication, learning essential early communication skills such as looking at faces (eye contact), turn-taking and sharing attention. Early identification of hearing-impairment, with resultant earlier intervention, should help promote positive communication strategies between parents and their deaf infants. However, many deaf toddlers and even school-aged children do present with problems in these areas – poor or avoidant eye contact, limited use of natural gesture or unwillingness or inability to focus on shared, adult-directed activity. One of the questions frequently asked of the psychologist is whether these difficulties are indicative of a communication disorder, or the result of an impoverished early communication experience. This will be explored fully in Chapter 5 in this book.

LANGUAGE

Children with a bilateral, severe or profound hearing loss do not generally develop oral language spontaneously because they cannot hear the language spoken naturally around them. The impact of deafness on language development is complex; many factors interact to produce the level of language attainment seen in any individual child. The aetiology of deafness and hence the quality of the auditory signal, the age at which the hearing loss is identified and appropriate aids fitted, the language input available before and after optimal aiding, the child's intellectual ability and familial and educational factors all combine to influence language development. In addition, the receptive and expressive components of deaf children's language development should be considered independently. Their ability to *understand* language may be very different from their ability to *produce* language, particularly spoken language. Even when a deaf child is considered 'oral', their intelligibility, expressive vocabulary and grammar skills may be extremely poor in relation to their hearing peers.

Considerable research has documented the impact of deafness on language development. For example, Davis *et al.* (1986) found that children with severe hearing losses (71–90dB) are more than three years behind their hearing peers in vocabulary development. Bishop (1983) showed that the comprehension of spoken vocabulary of profoundly deaf children between 8 and 12 years old, was less than that of hearing four-year-olds. Lederberg and Everhart (1998) found that by three years of age normally hearing children produce spoken sentences of several words, whereas deaf children are producing only occasional one-word utterances at the same age. This finding was independent of whether sign was used in addition to spoken language by the children's mothers.

In terms of grammar, deaf children's development is equally if not more delayed. The degree of difficulty a child experiences with learning English grammar when reading and writing appears to be positively related to the degree of hearing loss. Although deaf children may develop good language skills, both receptive and expressive, through sign language, the reading and writing skills of these children typically remain significantly delayed, possibly because sign languages have different grammar and syntax to that of English.

There are a number of clinical implications of these observations. For example, when communicating with a deaf child it is essential to take into account his or her level of language, particularly in terms of understanding vocabulary and the complexity of sentence structure. Discussions involving the child, explanations regarding the purpose of sessions, information and instructions for tests, will all need to be simplified by the psychologist to ensure full understanding by the child. Also, when assessing the cognitive abilities of a deaf child, it must be recognized that his or her language ability, or verbal intelligence is very unlikely to be a good indicator of his or her general intellectual ability, and therefore different assessment tools will be required (see Chapter 4 for detailed consideration of this topic).

TO SIGN OR NOT TO SIGN?

One of the major decisions facing parents of a child diagnosed with a significant, permanent hearing loss is whether or not to use sign language to communicate with them. Parents may receive widely differing and conflicting information and advice from different professionals and be left feeling angry, confused and helpless. In order for a sign language such as BSL to be acquired as a full complex language, like spoken language, it needs to develop from the infant's earliest days. Whilst sign language can be taught to older children and adults, more often than not this is not true BSL, but rather Sign Supported English (SSE), where the signs from BSL are used to accompany key words in speech using English rather than BSL grammar and syntax. When BSL is a first language, used from birth, usually by deaf parents of deaf children, research has shown that the language acquired is spontaneous and BSL grammar is learnt by the age of around five to six years (Chamberlain, Morford and Mayberry 2000). The older a child is when they start to learn sign language, the poorer their vocabulary, comprehension and accuracy. This supports the idea of a 'critical' period for language acquisition in early childhood.

Parents may be advised, or decide, to 'wait and see' whether their child develops adequate oral language, before adopting sign language. Clearly this may result in the child having very poor spoken language skills, and also severely delayed sign language skills. Many parents in the past have also been told that if they use signs with their deaf child, this will make their child 'lazy' in terms of their need or desire to use and develop spoken language. Thankfully there is no sound basis for this (in fact, there is evidence to the contrary – that having a language base through sign can act as a 'stepping stone' or frame on which to 'hang' spoken language development). Whilst it is essential for deaf children to have access to spoken language models and instruction for them to develop optimally using this mode, using sign language will not *prevent* this from happening. What is important, as Mayberry (2002) points out, is that exposure to language, be it signed or spoken, in early childhood, is essential for a first language to develop fully. Subsequently a second language can also be acquired, and the child can achieve grammatical and reading skills comparable to hearing children. In contrast, where there is no accessible language at the time when language is normally acquired (i.e. neither signed nor spoken) permanent deficits in language development result.

Since at least 90 per cent, and probably more than 95 per cent, of deaf children have hearing parents (Mitchell and Karchmer 2002) it is unsurprising that the majority of deaf babies and pre-school children have very limited exposure to sign language, particularly if the diagnosis of deafness is late. Although families may be taught some signs by professionals in the pre-school years, the level of language input the child is receiving typically falls well below that provided by access to a full, natural language. The educational and social interaction consequences of this will be explored in the following sections.

School attainments of deaf children

Not surprisingly, the academic achievements of deaf and hard of hearing children vary enormously, even when those children with additional difficulties are excluded from samples. A strong predictor of academic success is the level of hearing loss, as is socioeconomic status (Geers and Moog 1989; Mayberry 2002), but even then there are always notable individual exceptions to the rule.

Much research has focused on the reading achievements of deaf children. One of the most frequently quoted findings in the literature is that the average deaf 16-year-old is able to read at the level of a hearing nine-year-old. Whilst this generalization has some validity, as with most generalizations, it obscures more than it informs us. To be more precise, reading ability is associated with the degree of hearing loss, with those children with the most severe losses faring worst. In addition, early access to language, whether it is signed or spoken, predicts better reading skills in later childhood (see Mayberry 2002 for a discussion of this area). However, deaf children of deaf parents still do not typically achieve levels of literacy competence that match hearing children of hearing parents. Although sign languages are full, natural languages, they do not use English grammar or syntax and are therefore not an optimal basis for learning to read and write.

It might be expected that with the rise in the number of children receiving cochlear implants, resulting in better access to speech in the most significantly hearing-impaired, so too would there be a rise in literacy attainments amongst deaf children. Thoutenhoofd (2006) reports data from 152 implanted children that suggest that children with implants do indeed show greater educational attainments (reading, writing and mathematics) compared with non-implanted peers. However, there remains a gap between the achievements of this group and their hearing peers.

Social skills, peer interactions and friendships

The social interactions between children during early childhood are considered critical for the development of play skills, friendships and social competence, the last of which has implications for their socialization in the adult world. Given the language and communication delays so common amongst deaf children, social interactions are very often negatively impacted (see Antia and Kriemeyer 2003 for a review of the research literature in this area). They note that the frequency, duration and quality of interactions of deaf pre-school children with both deaf and hearing peers are all potentially affected by the child's language and communication skills. They also conclude that deaf children interact less frequently and for less time than do hearing peers, and engage more in solitary play and less in cooperative play. However, in general, deaf children with better language skills interact more than those with poor language skills.

Research has also suggested that deaf children try to initiate interactions just as frequently as their hearing peers, if not more so, and use similar initiation strategies but with different frequency. Unfortunately, deaf children's attempts may be more likely to be rejected, especially by their hearing peers. Martin and Bat-Chava (2003) examined the coping strategies of 5–11-year-old children in mainstream schools in terms of making friends with their hearing peers. They found gender differences such that in girls, confidence, willingness to ask for frequent clarification and being comfortable playing alone were associated with good relationships with hearing peers, whereas in boys it was the ability to perform well at sports that conferred an advantage. Finally, the themes of communication during social play appear to differ between deaf and hearing children such that the pretend play of deaf pre-schoolers tends to focus on literal or familiar events, in contrast to the fantasy themes commonly enjoyed by hearing children of this age.

Clearly, the situation is more complex than this brief summary suggests – other factors such as the setting in which they are observed, the communication mode of the dyad and the familiarity of the pair comprising the dyad all influence social interaction and play. The long-term consequences of these early differences can only be guessed at, and it is impossible to determine the exact influence of such early experiences. However, it is quite conceivable that self-esteem, self-confidence, mental health and educational and employment success are all impacted in some way.

Transitions

All children experience transitions during their formative years. These may range from moving house to the birth of a sibling, starting nursery school to reaching puberty. Hearing-impaired children, like their hearing peers, will vary in their reactions to significant changes in their lives depending on their temperament, previous experience of change, preparation for the event and many other factors.

For deaf children, certain transitions can be particularly difficult, and, as with so many of the challenges facing them, communicative competence is of great importance. Two of the most significant transitions for deaf and hard of hearing children are the moves from the home environment to nursery/pre-school or school, and the transition from junior/primary school to senior or secondary education. To our knowledge, there is no research literature looking at how deaf children cope with these moves. However, clinically we have found these to be triggers for referral for psychological help, or form a significant part of the history of emotional or behavioural problems presenting at a later point in time. At the younger age, of around three to four years, children may have had little experience of interacting with other children in groups. They may have great difficulty communicating with their hearing peers, experiencing isolation if not overt rejection. Even when they have deaf peers within the group and communication support from teaching or support staff (e.g. sign), some deaf children struggle to adjust to the demands of the classroom. They may resist conforming to the new routines of the setting or simply not understand what the desired behaviours are. This may result in a referral for behaviour problems.

The next major educational transition all children must negotiate is the move from primary to secondary education. In many ways this is more challenging than starting school, especially for deaf children. Primary schools are typically much smaller than secondary schools, with perhaps 200–300 pupils compared with up to 1800. In primary school, children usually have one main class teacher each year who they can get to know well, facilitating communication and understanding. In contrast, in secondary school, children have different teachers for each subject, all with different styles of communication, lip-patterns and accents to learn to follow. Also, many deaf children attend primary schools with specialist hearing-impaired 'units', where they spend significant proportions of their time in very small groups with the other deaf children or in one-to-one teaching. Thus, at the primary school level, deaf children are often empowered to develop a sense of security, mastery and positive self-esteem.

However, these very small deaf peer groups may work to the child's disadvantage in the transition process. Often a deaf child will be the only one in their year group, and the primary school where their hearing-impaired unit is located may not be a 'feeder' school for the secondary school that has provision for deaf children. Therefore, they may not transfer to the same secondary school as any of their classmates, losing both their hearing and deaf peer group. This makes it necessary for them to make new friends amongst a very large group of children where strong friendships are already established. Difficulties are often compounded by the deaf child's problems with communicating.

Another issue to be carefully considered when choosing appropriate secondary provision is the child's specific learning needs. Many deaf children have difficulties affecting academic progress in addition to the language deficits directly attributable to the deafness – dyslexia, attention problems, auditory-processing problems or language disorders (rather then simply delay). In the primary school setting they may receive more one-to-one specialist teaching than is available to children in the secondary school setting.

Psychological input for the child before and during this transition may involve assessing their learning ability and establishing any areas of specific difficulty, along with assessment of their social and emotional needs. Advice from a psychologist may be sought by the child's parents and/or teachers when considering options for secondary education. Sometimes problems arise once the secondary transfer has taken place, for example if the child struggles academically in the face of increased linguistic demands or has difficulty 'fitting in' with his or her new peer group. Clinically, children may present with behaviour problems, low mood or withdrawal, or symptoms of anxiety.

Cognitive consequences of childhood deafness

This topic is so broad in its scope and so complex that this section can only serve as the most elementary of introductions, highlighting the main issues. The interested reader is directed to look at book chapters by Mayberry (2002), Marschark (2003) and Edwards (2004) for further information, some of which is mentioned below.

Almost a century of research has yielded a wealth of findings from which a number of patterns are emerging, despite some conflicting results. In the past, differences between deaf and hearing individuals have typically been interpreted as deficits. More recently, with a greater understanding of cognitive processes generally and a wider range of test paradigms available to investigate them, research has produced some replicable results, which suggest that deafness per se does not typically make deaf children less cognitively able than their hearing peers. Rather, the absence of auditory stimulation may lead to changes in the way in which function is organized within the brain. The only robust finding that could be interpreted as a deficit is in short-term memory for auditory-verbal material, for example, the digit span test, which was first demonstrated by Pintner and colleagues as early as 1917 and has been much replicated since. Other areas that have been investigated include visual processing and attention, visual imagery (e.g. mental rotation tasks), visual short-term memory, working memory, semantic memory, problem-solving (e.g. analogical problems), other higher order and executive functions such as theory of mind, and, of course, IQ.

A number of factors are likely to influence deaf children's information-processing strategies and cognitive abilities. Arguably the most important is access to a full language from infancy, and hence the development of good language skills. The nature of that language is also important (i.e. signed versus spoken) in terms of the relationship between auditory deprivation and cognitive functioning.

Clinical psychologists need to have a good understanding of the cognitive abilities of deaf children for two main reasons. First, a significant proportion of referrals to a clinical psychologist are requests for an assessment of the child's cognitive abilities, or more particularly areas of specific difficulty. This is such an important area that a full chapter is devoted to the topic later in the book (Chapter 4). Second, in all interactions with a deaf child it is essential that the psychologist takes into account the intellectual abilities of the child as well as his or her language abilities as mentioned previously, tailoring language use to the specific abilities and needs of the child, to maximize comprehension.

Parenting and behaviour

The importance of effective communication with a deaf child for promoting positive behaviours should be readily apparent from previous sections. Once infants are mobile and able to explore their surroundings actively, the issues of boundary-setting and discipline become increasingly pertinent. There is substantial literature on the impact on parents of having a deaf child, for example in terms of parental stress and coping, parental roles in promoting communication and language, parent–professional roles and family functioning. However, relatively little has focused directly on the practical aspects of parenting a deaf child. The National Deaf Children's Society (NDCS) commissioned and published a psychosocial literature-based review of parenting and deaf children (NDCS 2003a), which was followed by a Needs Assessment of this group, resulting in the development of a 'Parents' Toolkit'. The work highlights the tension between being a 'normal' mum or dad, doing the things parents typically do with their children, and performing roles most parents do not have to engage in – being their child's teacher, therapist, advocate and technology expert.

The NDCS Needs Assessment (NDCS 2003b), in which over 1300 parents of deaf children contributed to findings through in-depth interviews and questionnaires, highlights a number of similarities and differences in parenting a deaf child compared with a hearing one, and the skills and personal attributes needed to parent successfully. The study explored a wide variety of factors that may influence parenting attitudes, including whether the child has additional disabilities, previous parenting experience, the severity of deafness, the age of the child and the hearing status of the parents. The results are highly complex, and this brief summary cannot begin to do justice to the richness and importance of the findings, which have immense relevance to psychologists and other professionals working with deaf children and families. Characteristics that were identified as being necessary and helpful in parenting a deaf child included perseverance, patience, assertiveness, being articulate, tolerating uncertainty, learning to take control and becoming 'braver', and believing in one's own ability. Parenting issues that were generally perceived as being difficult with a deaf child included warning of danger, managing frustration, dealing with emotions, communication, building the child's confidence and mixing with other children.

As a result of the myriad of possible combinations of factors outlined in the above sections (responses to diagnosis, communication and language, social development and friendships, cognitive ability and parenting) it is not surprising that at times things go awry. Emotional or behavioural problems may be the consequence of and are frequently the catalyst for referral of a deaf child to mental health or psychology services. Deaf children are at greater risk of psychological and psychiatric disorders than their hearing peers (e.g. Hindley 1997; Hindley *et al.* 1994), and yet are significantly disadvantaged in terms of their access to appropriate services. This area will be explored in depth in the next chapter.

Siblings

As we saw in earlier sections, the impact on hearing parents of having a deaf child is usually profound, influencing the family dynamics and sometimes putting a strain on the parents' relationship. Despite this there is currently no research specifically exploring the relationship between deaf children and their hearing siblings, or evaluating the consequences for the hearing child of having a deaf sibling. In contrast, a considerable body of research has accumulated on the impact on well siblings of having a sibling with a disability, and this literature can provide useful insights for our work with deaf children and their siblings.

Stoneman (2005) reviews the research findings in this area. She points out that despite the assumption underlying much of the research that having a sibling with a disability must be bad for children, many studies have found no evidence for negative effects on self-concept, perceived competence, behaviour, loneliness or self-efficacy. Indeed, having a sibling with a disability may result in higher internal locus of control and less sibling conflict, and positive, nurturing relationships between the siblings.

However, there is evidence that a small proportion of children are adversely affected, exhibiting emotional or behaviour problems particularly when the disability in the sibling is severe. A number of factors have been proposed as possible predictors of adjustment problems. These include stress associated with the sibling relationship itself and stress arising from events occurring in the family environment, both directly and indirectly relating to the child with the disability. For example, Giallo and Gavidia-Payne (2006) found that socioeconomic status, past attendance at a sibling support group, parental stress, family routines, family problem-solving skills and family hardiness significantly predicted sibling adjustment problems. Interestingly, the siblings' own experience of stress and the coping strategies they used were not associated with adjustment. Williams *et al.* (2002) also found that socioeconomic status and family cohesion were significant predictors of well-sibling behaviour problems. Other important factors in the adjustment of the well sibling were their knowledge of their sibling's disability or illness, self-esteem and their perception of the social support they receive from parents, teachers, close friends and classmates.

Whatever the reality of the manner in which parents behave towards their deaf children compared with hearing siblings, deaf children may feel that they are treated differently, or believe that their parents love their hearing siblings more. It may be that parents really do have different expectations regarding acceptable behaviour, or give their deaf child more attention, for example because they have to attend so many appointments or work with them on listening or language activities. This may lead to strong feelings of jealousy and then guilt or shame, or overt sibling rivalry. Glover (2003) reflects on her personal experience of raising three sons, two of whom have a profound hearing loss. She describes the joy the elder of the two deaf boys expressed on learning that his baby brother was also deaf, and also the stress of coping with constant fighting between the boys. Woolfe (2001) interviewed deaf children with deaf siblings and deaf children with hearing siblings (with either hearing or deaf parents) and found that even when children had a deaf sibling, they experienced frustration and jealousy when communicative competence and speech skills differed between them. This was even more pronounced when the deaf child had a hearing sibling, and was associated with low self-esteem, anxiety and ambivalent or even hostile feelings. One child felt that his hearing brother was embarrassed by him, resulting in the hearing brother refusing to allow his deaf sibling join in with him and his friends.

These findings highlight a number of areas that could form the focus of therapeutic work with deaf children, their parents and siblings. One of the most important lessons to be learned from the findings is that the most effective input is likely to be the need to focus on the whole family rather than any one individual. Improvements in psychological well-being are likely to result from strategies that enhance the family's problem-solving and negotiating skills, along with shared decision-making and use of coping strategies. Intervention may involve helping parents to find and develop the most effective communication strategies between all members of the family, and to build strong family structures and routines, for example encouraging each child to take part in appropriate leisure activities. It is also very important to provide the hearing sibling(s) with information about deafness, and in particular the cause of deafness in their family (if known) as this can create considerable misunderstanding and anxiety. Throughout any intervention it is essential that the therapist is mindful of factors that influence psychological well-being in the children but over which the parents may have little or no control, for example financial stresses, inadequate or poor housing and difficulties attending multiple appointments often at great distances from their home.

Working therapeutically with deaf children and their families

Psychological services specifically designed to meet the needs of deaf children in the UK are few and far between. Often it is only those children with the most severe difficulties who receive help, and most will have to travel long distances to access it. Families often feel very isolated when experiencing difficulties, as they perceive their child to be different from other children with seemingly similar problems, and this feeling may be reinforced when local child and adolescent mental health services refuse to accept a referral for input, arguing that the child requires specialist input from teams experienced in working with deaf individuals. Although a number of policy documents recommend improving the accessibility of specialist services (e.g. NIMHE/DH 2005), it is possible for non-specialist services to provide appropriate interventions given support and advice from professionals experienced in the field.

The preceding descriptions of the impact of deafness on a child and his or her family will have given a flavour of the kinds of issues that are of relevance when conducting an initial assessment of a deaf child referred for psychological input. Formulation of the problem(s) will need to include all the traditional factors, plus those more specific to the experience of deafness.

Although there are probably more similarities than differences in the way in which a psychologist may work therapeutically with a deaf child compared with a hearing one, there are a number of practical issues that it is essential to address for any interaction or intervention to be effective. The room in which the child is seen is of great importance. It needs to be well lit, so that the child can see the psychologist's face clearly to aid lip-reading and reading facial expressions, and should be carpeted and curtained to reduce background noise from sounds bouncing off hard surfaces. Lip-reading is obviously only possible if the child can see the therapist's mouth clearly, so it is important to avoid covering the mouth with the hands whilst speaking. Eye contact is crucial, so unlike some therapeutic situations where the therapist sits diagonally from the client, it is better for them to sit directly opposite. However, being too close is not helpful – around one to two metres apart is best. As with most children, it is wise to make sure you have their full attention before trying to talk (or sign) to them – this may need to be achieved by tapping them on the arm, or even gently raising their chin to make sure they are looking at you. However, some deaf children find this intrusive, so care must be taken to check with parents that this is a method the child is used to and finds acceptable. Even if a deaf child does not use sign language it is still very helpful to use gestures and facial expressions to aid understanding, for example to show when a question is being asked, or to convey emotions. If there are a number of people in the room, for example the child's parents and other professionals, it is important that only one person speaks at a time, and that sufficient time is allowed for the child to understand what one person has said before the next one starts. New topics of conversation need to be clearly indicated, so that the child can follow what is being said, in order to encourage their full participation. Any child who feels that they are being 'left out' or misunderstood will have little incentive to try to communicate and participate fully in the session. Modelling positive interactions and communication strategies by the therapist can be an important part of the therapeutic process, potentially eliminating the necessity for explicitly pointing out ways in which the communication of family members is problematic.

Conclusions

At first reckoning it might be assumed that being deaf would have little impact on the development of a child, beyond preventing the normal acquisition of speech and language skills. Whilst it is true that hearing impairment may have a disastrous impact on the development of language, and in some children communication generally, the reality is that the consequences go far beyond this, and are far more complex. Many factors determine the child's acquisition of language and communication, including whether they have any disabilities in addition to their deafness, the age at which they were diagnosed, communication choices made by their parents, schooling and many more besides. The child's ability to communicate effectively with their family, peers and members of the wider community, and be understood in return, is of fundamental importance in determining their psychological well-being, both during childhood and beyond. Where difficulties arise, for example in terms of emotional or behavioural problems, it is essential that these are recognized, acknowledged and addressed in a timely, appropriate fashion by professionals who feel competent to deal with deafness as part of the presenting concerns of the child and family.

2 Behavioural and Emotional Disorders

In this chapter we will consider a wide range of problems faced by many families of deaf children, and people involved in their care, including their teachers and other professionals. We have used the words 'behavioural and emotional disorders' in the chapter heading and this requires some clarification. Depending on the viewpoint of the individual practitioner or researcher and the context within which they are working, 'emotional/behavioural disorders' may mean very different things. Broadly speaking, it is possible to think about this group of problems from two perspectives – the medical or psychiatric model, or a more general psychological approach. In the former, the emphasis is on diagnosis of specific disorders or conditions, such as conduct disorder, autism, oppositional disorder, depression, childhood schizophrenia, obsessive-compulsive disorder, anorexia nervosa or attention deficit hyperactivity disorder (ADHD), using clearly defined criteria. Given the low incidence of permanent childhood deafness, combined with the low rates of some of these disorders in the hearing population during childhood (e.g. schizophrenia) it is not surprising that most professionals working in the mental health field, or indeed education or social services, will not have come across a deaf child diagnosed with one of these disorders. In contrast, the majority of professionals who work with deaf children will be able to identify children they have seen where behaviour is a significant issue resulting in disruption to the child's development, family functioning and later on, schooling. Included in this group of 'disorders', which are most common amongst pre-school children, are sleep problems, eating problems, toileting difficulties, temper tantrums, hearing-device (non-)compliance and attention problems. In older children, problems of anxiety, depression or self-esteem are more common, and may result in referral to school counselling or local child and adolescent mental health services. For the remainder of this chapter we will use the term 'behavioural disorders' to encompass those conditions that have well-defined diagnostic criteria and labels, for example ADHD, and 'behaviour problems' for those that are more nebulous, such as general compliance and temper tantrum problems in a toddler.

The focus of this chapter will be on those behavioural disorders and problems that are most frequently encountered by anyone involved with deaf children, regardless of whether they are traditionally viewed within a medical model, although other disorders may also be briefly considered. The chapter will start with some statistics on the prevalence of behavioural disorders, and the difficulties in accurately determining this. Reasons why deaf children are at particular risk for developing behaviour problems will be explored, as this provides valuable insights into useful intervention strategies. This will be followed by discussion of psychological assessment and formulation, and treatment approaches.

Epidemiology

Assessing and diagnosing behavioural disorders or problems in hearing-impaired children is fraught with difficulties. Several studies over the past 30 years or so have attempted to determine prevalence rates for behaviour disorders amongst deaf children and adolescents. The first challenge when trying to interpret the findings of such studies is in the terminology used. Phrases such as 'psychiatric disorder', 'psychiatric disturbance', 'behaviour disorder', 'mental health problem' and 'behavioural and emotional problem' abound, and many are used inconsistently within the same study. Second, the assessment methods used also vary widely, making it difficult to interpret or generalize findings. This said, some consistency of findings is emerging. Freeman, Malkin and Hastings (1975) and Fundudis, Kolvin and Garside (1979) used combinations of questionnaire measures, interviews and child observation and reported elevated rates of disturbance compared with hearing norms or controls, with a prevalence rate of up to 54 per cent in one group of deaf children. However, early studies can be criticized for using questionnaires not validated for hearing-impaired children (including, for example, speech-related items, which are clearly inappropriate for many deaf children), and for not interviewing the children themselves. This may have led to the greater number of 'conduct' type disorders identified in comparison with emotional or affective disorders in some studies.

More recently, Hindley *et al.* (1994) described the development of a screening instrument specifically for use with culturally Deaf children, and used this to estimate the prevalence of psychiatric disorder in 11–16-year-old children attending a Deaf School compared with those in hearing-impaired units (HIUs). Importantly, the questionnaires were followed by interviews with the children conducted with sign language interpreters. They reported prevalence rates of 42.4 per cent and 60.9 per cent in the Deaf Schools and HIUs respectively, with a relative paucity of depressive disorders and excess of social phobias compared with the general population. Vostanis *et al.* (1997) compared rates of emotional and behavioural problems identified by two questionnaire measures, both completed by the parents of 84 children with pre-lingual severe to profound deafness. The first, the Child Behaviour Checklist (CBCL; Achenbach 1991a, 1992) is a widely used instrument, with versions for children from 2 to 18 years of age. The second measure, the Parent's Checklist (PCL), was developed specifically for deaf children (Hindley *et al.* 1994). According to the CBCL, 40 per cent of the sample could be considered to have clinically significant problems, whilst the PCL identified 77 per cent of the children as having emotional or behavioural disorders.

Notably, none of the above studies report prevalence rates for specific diagnoses such as obsessive-compulsive disorder or anorexia nervosa. However, there is some evidence from other studies regarding the rate of ADHD or hyperkinetic disorder amongst deaf children. As usual, differing terminology, diagnostic criteria and practices, particularly between the UK and USA, make it difficult to draw any firm conclusions. This said, it is widely accepted that hearing-impaired children are more prone to problems with attention control and/or hyperactivity than their hearing peers, and evidence suggests that such problems are more associated with acquired deafness (congenital rubella, congenital cytomegalovirus and meningitis) and consequent generalized brain abnormalities than with deafness per se (Kelly *et al.* 1993). For a full discussion of the theoretical and epidemiological aspects of attention deficit and overactivity in deaf children, see Hindley and Kroll (1998).

Overall, bearing in mind differences in the definitions of disorders, differing sampling and assessment methodologies between studies and consequent huge variability in prevalence estimates, it appears that deaf children and adolescents are at greater risk than their hearing peers for psychosocial maladjustment in a general sense and behavioural disorders and problems specifically.

Why are deaf children at greater risk of behavioural disorders?

The complex links between language, cognition, social and emotional development have been much debated and theorized (e.g. Vygotsky 1986). In order to
understand the impact of hearing-impairment on the development of social and
emotional well-being, and hence mental health and behavioural disorders, it is
useful to consider first the relationship between language delay or disorders,
communication skills and behavioural problems. As Cohen (1996) notes, the
formation and maintenance of social relationships are related to language and
cognitive development, including the ability to use emotion labels to reflect on
and talk about feelings and understand the consequences of actions. Poor social
skills, which are likely in part to arise from poor language skills, may contribute
to the misinterpretation of the intentions and motives of other children, leading
to negative social interactions. For example, language-impaired children may
appear not to care about the impact of something they have said or done, or may
respond aggressively, because they have misunderstood the communication of
others.

Language delay has been found to be associated with overactivity, and
problems with soiling, wetting and dependency in children aged three years
(Stevenson and Richman 1978). Expressive language problems have been associated with distractibility, impulsivity and hyperactivity (Beitchman 1985).
Behaviour problems are typically found in around half of children with speech
and language delays. However, such problems may be more strongly related to
language disorders rather than simply delayed speech development.
School-aged children (aged 6–11 years) with language delay are described as
having low self-confidence, low self-esteem and being socially withdrawn
(Haynes and Naidoo 1991). It is interesting to note that problems indicating
high levels of frustration and aggression are more common in younger children
and tend to decline with time, whilst difficulties of a more socio-emotional
nature remain, or increase. Thus, Rutter and Mawhood (1991) conclude that the
predominant problems in later childhood are anxiety, social relationships and
attention deficits, rather than conduct disorders or anti-social behaviour.

A number of possible explanations for the association between language
delay and behaviour problems can be proposed. The first is that they have a
common aetiology, the most obvious being a genetic cause. An example of
possible shared aetiology is in dyslexia, which is frequently found together with
attention problems, suggesting there may be a common neurodevelopmental
precursor or deficit responsible for both. Other possible shared causes might

include parenting or socioeconomic factors. The next possibility is that language delay and behaviour problems may have separate causes but ones that are themselves correlated. Finally, language delay may lead to behavioural disorders, or vice-versa, or there may be a reciprocal relationship between the two. For example, deficits in the child's pragmatic understanding and use of language may lead to problems communicating effectively, which in turn lead to high levels of frustration, and problems such as aggressive behaviour, anxiety or social withdrawal. The child then has reduced opportunities for developing appropriate language skills from positive interactions with peers and adults. Stevenson (1996) provides a very helpful diagrammatic conceptualization of the possible aetiological mechanisms for co-morbid language disorder and behaviour problems from a developmental perspective.

Observation of the links between communication, socio-emotional development and behaviour in deaf children has led to one of the few interventions specifically designed for deaf children: 'Promoting Alternative Thinking Strategies', or PATHS®. Greenberg and Kusché (1998) implemented this school-based preventative intervention aimed at improving children's behavioural adjustment including self-control, increased emotional understanding and social problem-solving skills. A waiting-list control design was used, such that half the sample received the intervention during the first year of the study, and the remainder received it during the second year. The authors report that the PATHS® curriculum was effective in improving affective and social cognitive understanding, social competence and behaviour, along with improvements in parent and teacher ratings of child psychopathology in the second group of children, for whom the curriculum had been revised following feedback from the teachers of the first group. Improvements were maintained at two years post-intervention.

In a smaller-scale study, Dyck and Denver (2003) evaluated the effectiveness of an educational programme, 'The Funny Faces Program', designed to enhance the ability of deaf children to understand their own and others' emotional experiences. They did not include a control group, and post-intervention measures were obtained within two weeks of the end of the programme – no further follow-up is reported. However, significant increases in emotion vocabulary and emotion comprehension were observed, with those children with moderate to severe hearing losses (but not profound) showing equivalent emotion recognition abilities to their hearing peers at the end of the programme.

Communication, deafness and behavioural disorders

It is not difficult to see the relevance of these findings to the hearing-impaired child. Whilst only a minority of deaf children are diagnosed as having a language disorder, the majority of deaf children have some degree of language delay, for many of whom the delay is severe. The association between the quality and effectiveness of communication between deaf children and their parents and socio-emotional development is complex, and includes implications for social behaviour (see Vaccari and Marschark 1997 for a discussion of this area). Musselman *et al.* (1996) report the findings of a study of communicative competence and psychosocial development in deaf children, first assessing them when aged around six years, and then again in adolescence, aged 16 years. All the children had hearing losses in the severe to profound range, were pre-lingually deafened and had hearing parents. Their non-verbal IQ averaged 108. Ninety per cent of the sample were receiving auditory/oral education after diagnosis of their hearing impairment. However, by the end of the pre-school phase of the study (i.e. aged six years) only 60 per cent remained in oral education, and by adolescence this was reduced further to 33 per cent. The remainder had moved to Total Communication (TC) approaches. Communicative competence was divided into speech skills and comprehension, both of which were significantly delayed compared with hearing norms in early childhood. Psychosocial development was assessed by parent interview, and addressed self-help skills, social relations (sleep, play, peer relationships) and social comprehension (personal space, responsibility and functional sequences). At age six years there was some evidence for a relationship between communicative competence and both social relations and social comprehension in those children who communicated orally. In the TC group, spoken language skills were not related to psychosocial development, but a strong relationship was found between language comprehension and all the social development indices. In adolescence, the TC group was found to be experiencing more internalizing and externalizing behaviour problems (somatic complaints, anxiety/depression, social problems, attention problems and aggressive behaviour) than the group that was still being educated aurally/orally. However, in the TC group, psychosocial problems were not related to communicative competence. Interestingly, there was a significant association between language comprehension scores at age six years, and both internalizing and externalizing problems in adolescence such that superior early language skills are associated with better adjustment in adolescence.

A more recent study by Wallis, Musselman and MacKay (2004) supports the importance of effective early communication for later psychological well-being amongst deaf adolescents. They compared 15 signing deaf children of hearing parents where exposure to sign language commenced early in life and was consistent throughout childhood, with 27 whose exposure to sign started later and whose mothers did not sign. They also included a group of 15 deaf children exposed to aural/oral communication throughout childhood. A version of the Youth Self-report questionnaire (YSF; Achenbach 1991b) adapted for deaf adolescents was administered. The highest rates of clinical 'caseness' were found in the 'late' signing group and the lowest in the aural/oral group, with the 'early' signing group in between, although the difference between the latter two groups was not significant. Combining the early signing and aural/oral groups revealed significantly fewer mental health problems compared with the later signers. The results support the idea that an early and consistent communication mode match between deaf children and their hearing mothers is important for future mental health.

As we saw in Chapter 1 of this book, hearing-impairment can have a profound impact on a child's development of language, cognitive skills and on their school achievements, social skills and ability to form friendships. Their ability to understand what they are being asked to do, how to do it and the consequences of their actions may be severely impaired. Thus, it should come as no surprise that hearing-impaired children are at risk for developing a wide range of behavioural disorders or problems. The one theme that underpins all the above issues is that of the essentiality of effective communication, between deaf children and their parents especially, but also their peers and the wider community. Therefore, this is a thread that will be seen to run throughout the remainder of this chapter.

Common behavioural disorders in deaf children

In this section we will briefly describe the most commonly presenting behaviour problems and disorders and explore the impact of deafness on their presentation.

Temper tantrums

Temper tantrums are a normal, if challenging part of the early years of most children. Tantrums are most common between one and three years of age and vary in intensity and duration, from a few minutes' whining or crying to an extended period of kicking, screaming, hitting and breath-holding. Tantrums occur when toddlers are unable to control or master their environment, when they can't have or do what they want, or want attention, and are more likely to happen when the child is tired, hungry or uncomfortable. The tantrum 'phase' in deaf toddlers often lasts longer and the tantrums are more frequent and intense than in their hearing counterparts. Tantrums are most common during the second year of life when children are typically rapidly acquiring language, but are able to understand more than they can express. Given the language delay of most deaf children it should be predicted that many become frustrated and have tantrums when they cannot communicate what they are thinking or feeling, or feel confused, or don't understand what they are expected to do or why.

In deaf children, tantrums often present in the context of severe difficulties for the parents in setting and enforcing appropriate behavioural boundaries, with consequent generalized problems of non-compliance in the child. Many parents express their feelings of helplessness in communicating instructions and explanations to their child, sometimes to the point where they give up trying. There is some research evidence that mothers of children with profound hearing losses are more likely to use physical discipline in response to unwanted behaviours than mothers of hearing children (Knutson, Johnson and Sullivan 2004), and this is certainly our impression clinically.

Toileting problems

This area of difficulty is not one that naturally springs to mind in the context of hearing-impairment. However, it is included here because of the frequency with which we have encountered requests for help with this issue from parents of hearing-impaired children. Bladder control typically starts to become attainable from around a child's second birthday and bowel control sometime after that, but there is huge variability in when parents choose to start the process of toilet training, and how long it takes to become fully established. If a child is not toilet-trained by around four years of age, it suggests that there is an issue that needs to be resolved, either with the child or the parents. It is important to make sure that there is no medical reason why it has not been possible for the child to gain bladder and/or bowel control, before looking for psychological explanations, and therefore we would always recommend that the child is seen by their general practitioner or paediatrician, as appropriate. It appears that if toilet training is not accomplished during the period when the child is developmentally ready, then using a nappy becomes a 'habit' that the child is reluctant to give up. The longer they continue to use one, the harder it is for them to learn to use the toilet. It is our clinical impression that a significant proportion of deaf children become toilet-trained at a later age than their hearing peers. Sometimes parents of deaf children say that they just 'haven't got around to' starting toilet training because of the many other demands on them in terms of caring for a deaf child. Others feel unable to explain to their child what they want them to do, or get into battles with their child over 'performing' in the right place. Unfortunately this is one battle parents can never win! Others again have expressed their uncertainty over whether their child should be expected to learn to use the toilet at the typical age, given the many challenges they face in mastering the communication and language skills appropriate for their age. Generally we find that as long as children do not have any additional disabilities, they can master toileting at the same time as their hearing peers with appropriate parental support.

Sleep problems

Difficulties achieving good sleeping patterns amongst babies and toddlers are extremely common: around a third of infants and toddlers are described by their parents as having a sleep problem (e.g. Bayer *et al.* 2007), and such problems have been linked to poorer maternal health and well-being. In pre-school children, sleep problems are associated with behaviour problems, attention and hyperactivity problems and poorer quality of life (Hiscock *et al.* 2007). In deaf children, sleep problems also frequently present in the context of generalized behavioural problems, difficulties with setting appropriate boundaries and poor parent–child communication. The types of sleep problems encountered in deaf children are the same as those in hearing children – difficulties getting the child to settle at an appropriate bedtime in their own bed, trouble achieving sleep independently (i.e. the child will only fall asleep if being cuddled by a parent or with a parent lying beside them), frequent waking during the night and entering the parent's bed during the night. Deaf children also sometimes present with a pattern of behaviour suggestive of night terrors. In addition, deaf children may exhibit signs of anxiety or fear around going to bed, which may be linked to difficulties communicating in a darkened room. As with other behaviour problems, parents of deaf children often say that it is not possible to explain to their toddler what they want them to do, or may feel that it is 'unfair' to impose rules on their child when they already have so many obstacles to overcome in their everyday lives. Young deaf children do indeed frequently have difficulty with concepts such as later, next, quickly, if and when. However, many behaviour problems often arise simply as the result of the under-use of clear, consistently enforced boundaries and the word 'no', which it is quite possible to convey to a very young deaf child with no room for misunderstanding!

Hearing-aid compliance

Although lack of compliance with recommended use of a medical device is not traditionally considered either a behavioural disorder or behaviour problem, it is included here as it is a very common presenting problem to professionals working with hearing-impaired children.

Most children with a moderate hearing loss or greater will be issued with hearing aids. With the advent of the Newborn Hearing Screening Programme in the UK and elsewhere, hearing aids may first be fitted when an infant is only a few weeks old. When this is the case, if parents are committed to their use, the infant typically accepts the aids without difficulty, and they become part of the child's 'clothing'. However, hearing loss can occur at any age, and therefore hearing aids may need to be first worn when the child is in the middle of the 'terrible twos' and wearing the aids may become one of the few aspects of the child's life over which they have control. Pulling the hearing aids out, dismantling them, throwing them into the road or down the toilet is usually a very effective means of gaining attention or demonstrating anger or frustration, or an indication that the child is unsettled in some way. It is not uncommon for children to present with a history of general non-compliance with refusal to wear their hearing aids as one of the behaviours their parents find most challenging. Toddlers can become extremely adept at pulling one hearing aid out as their mother struggles to put the other one in, so that much of the day is spent simply trying to replace them.

Parents, and indeed some professionals working with deaf children and their families, may be ambivalent about the usefulness of wearing hearing aids, and this may be conveyed to the child in a number of ways. It may be that the child is only asked to wear the aids when at nursery, or when attending audiological clinic appointments, or the parents may convey through their body language that they lack confidence in putting the aids in and are not willing to risk upsetting the child or provoking a tantrum. It is also sometimes the case that parents have not come to terms with their child's deafness, and this is influencing their attitude towards hearing-aid use.

Obsessive-compulsive disorder

Obsessive-compulsive disorder (OCD) is a behaviour disorder that has been estimated to affect 0.25 per cent of UK 5–15-year-olds (Heyman *et al.* 2001), but almost nothing is written about with regard to deaf children or adolescents. OCD can start at any age but most commonly starts during childhood or adolescence and may co-exist with other disorders such as autism, ADHD, depression or anxiety. Obsessions are thoughts that the person is unable to stop occurring and that happen over and over again, and which usually cause anxiety or distress. For example, the child may be unable to stop thinking about something bad happening or what comes next in their school timetable. The obsessions experienced by deaf children may be subtly different from those of hearing children. They may focus more on schedules or what is going to happen next, rather than fears about germs or hurting someone. A deaf child with a problem of this sort can be very hard to identify if he or she does not have the language to tell the therapist about it. However, if the child is able to describe his or her thoughts, careful questioning can elicit whether the thoughts are in response to difficulties in communication or in understanding something, resulting in the need to keep going over a topic until they feel sure that they fully understand, or whether they are unrelated to current events, are intrusive and not stopped by being given adequate information or reassurance.

Compulsions are behaviours that the individual needs to repeat over and over again, in order to reduce feelings of anxiety. Most compulsions appear irrational, for example touching something eight times before leaving the house, washing hands many many times or keeping empty shampoo bottles that are not needed. As with obsessions, the compulsions experienced by deaf children may differ from their hearing peers. For example, the child may need to repeat a particular sign over and over again, or ask the same question repeatedly despite receiving an answer he or she is able to understand linguistically.

Obsessive-compulsive disorder can be difficult to identify in deaf children, particularly those with poor language or communication skills. They are more likely to be seen as overly anxious or on the autistic spectrum of disorders, or simply have their 'strange' behaviour attributed to being deaf, rather than as having OCD.

Attention deficit hyperactivity disorder

Three main subtypes of attention deficit hyperactivity disorder (ADHD) are generally accepted – predominantly inattentive (attention deficit disorder; ADD); predominantly hyperactive (impulsive) and a mixed or combined subtype. The disorder is found in around 7–8 per cent of all children and is around three times more common in boys. Although approximately the same rates of the disorder are found in deaf children, many more, between 30 and 40 per cent, have some difficulties in maintaining appropriate classroom behaviour. Delays in language acquisition are associated with delays in the development of executive functions, with the result that deaf children are more likely to experience difficulties in mastering affect regulation (control of mood or emotions) and verbally mediated self-control, resulting in the behavioural manifestations of ADHD.

One of the main difficulties in identifying ADHD in deaf children is the overlap in behaviours considered diagnostic of ADHD and those common amongst deaf children. For example, the *DSM-IV* diagnostic criteria (American Psychiatric Association 1994) include behaviours such as 'Often does not seem to listen when spoken to directly', 'Is often forgetful in daily activities', 'Often has trouble organizing activities', 'Often interrupts or intrudes on others' and 'Often blurts out answers before questions have been finished'. A deaf child may not realize they are being spoken to, and may forget instructions because they have not fully understood them. They may also have difficulty organizing or completing tasks because they do not fully understand the written or oral instructions they have been given. They may appear very easily distracted by what is going on around them when in fact they are monitoring their environment to check who is talking, or to gain information. They may have difficulty sustaining attention, particularly on a teacher providing new or complex information orally, due to fatigue at having to concentrate so hard for an extended period. Similarly, in terms of problems with overactivity, the deaf child may seem unduly fidgety because they have become restless after concentrating for a long time on a verbal task. They may blurt out answers to questions before the question has been completed because they cannot clearly see the speaker's face and thought they had finished. Similarly, deaf children may appear to be interrupting or intruding on others' conversations, whereas in fact they may not realize that someone else is talking, or may have difficulty with pragmatic language skills.

Thus, differentiating true attention deficit and overactivity problems from behaviours associated with poor language or social skills in deaf children is not straightforward. However, it is slightly easier in terms of hyperactivity-impulsivity symptoms, as there are a number of these that are not typically associated with hearing impairment. For example, deaf children are no more likely to leave their seats in the classroom inappropriately, run or climb excessively, have difficulty playing quietly or waiting their turn than their hearing peers.

Oppositional defiant disorder

Oppositional defiant disorder (ODD) is a behavioural disorder characterized by angry outbursts, purposeful rule-breaking or disobedience and arguing 'for the sake of it'. It is one of the most common behavioural disorders of early and middle childhood, affecting more boys than girls. There appears to be a higher incidence amongst deaf children, but this is complicated by the fact that there is considerable overlap between the behaviours associated with ODD and those found in ADHD, autism spectrum disorders, anxiety and depression.

Angry outbursts in children and adolescents are a normal part of development but in children with ODD the problems are more intense, frequent and persistent. Whilst deaf children may have ODD, many have angry outbursts because they are frustrated at being unable to communicate effectively rather than as a result of ODD. Poor communication skills, especially with peers, may lead to problems with empathizing and social problem-solving, resulting in a lack of the skills needed to deal with situations where the deaf child may feel left out, misunderstood or foolish. Modelling of aggressive behaviours may have occurred within the family context during the child's early years, when parents of deaf children are more likely to have used physical discipline with their deaf child, as a result of difficulties communicating without a shared, fluent language.

Assessment

General considerations

Achieving an accessible, thorough, appropriate assessment for a hearing-impaired child suspected of having a behaviour disorder is currently a challenge for mental health services. Given the low incidence of deafness in the general population and the lack of specific training of mental health professionals in issues relating to deafness, it is unsurprising that many behaviour problems and disorders go undiagnosed in hearing-impaired children. In the UK there are a very limited number of supra-regional, highly specialist mental health services for deaf people, predominantly catering for culturally Deaf individuals, or BSL users. However, given that the vast majority of deaf children have two hearing parents, and do not become fluent BSL users, these services may not be perceived as appropriate for them, by both the families and professionals involved. It is possible that families experiencing significant behavioural problems in their hearing-impaired child will be referred to their local child and adolescent mental health services. Unfortunately it is our experience that such services frequently feel de-skilled when faced with a deaf child, particularly one who has limited communication skills in any mode, and are reluctant to take on the referral. Families also sometimes express reservations about seeing professionals who are not specialists in deafness, due to concerns that their child's problems will not be fully understood. Having said this, there are many commonalities between behaviour problems in deaf and hearing children, and in terms of their assessment, along with treatment approaches. Working with deaf children should not therefore be seen as solely the remit of highly specialist deaf services, but as part of the responsibility of all mental health services, but with support from, and the option of referral to such specialist services when appropriate.

When assessing a deaf child, one of the most important tasks is to ensure that as far as it is possible, the assessment is multi-disciplinary. If it is not possible to involve the relevant services or professionals in the assessment process at that time, it is essential that as much recent information is collated as possible, for example reports from the child's speech and language therapist, educational psychologist, paediatrician and the school or nursery. It is also essential to have up-to-date information on the extent and nature of the child's hearing loss. If recent, relevant information is not available it may be necessary to request assessments from these professionals. In particular it is very helpful to have an assessment of the child's language and communication abilities, and his or her cognitive/learning skills.

As with the assessment of any child presenting with behaviour problems, it is usually necessary to consider the difficulties in a variety of contexts, and therefore observation of the child at nursery or school, or at home in very young children is recommended.

Before the first interview the child's (and parent's) preferred mode of communication must be established so that a BSL interpreter can be booked if necessary. If there is any uncertainty about whether the child needs an interpreter it is better to err on the side of caution. If there is to be more than one assessment session it is helpful to have the same interpreter if at all possible, as they (and the interviewer) will benefit from the increased understanding of, and rapport they will have developed with the child, as the signs used by many children are not always accurately formed or placed, or may be used idiosyncratically, taking some time for the interpreter to become familiar with. When working with a sign language interpreter, consideration must be given to the extra time that will be needed for the interview and perhaps to de-brief the interpreter after the session. Adequate lighting must be ensured, and the interpreter and any other signers should not sit with their backs to a bright light source (e.g. window). The temptation to use parents or teachers as interpreters should be resisted, as they may misinterpret what the child is trying to say, be selective about what they interpret, or prevent the child from being able to disclose significant information. It is also not wise to assume that older children will be able to communicate in written form, as their literacy skills are likely to be delayed and prevent this from being an option.

Assessment – history

In addition to the traditional topics covered in the assessment of behavioural problems by a psychologist (description of the problem behaviours, when they started, precipitating and perpetuating factors and so on), there are a number of areas specific to deafness that should be explored. These are summarized below:

- issues around the diagnosis of deafness including:
  - age at diagnosis (congenital? progressive? suddenly acquired?)
  - family reactions to diagnosis, including extended family
  - how and by whom was the diagnosis given

- cause of deafness if known, and family history of hearing-impairment

- communication strategies and modes tried, and currently used by family members

- involvement with professionals and services

- additional disabilities

- cultural attitudes towards deafness (other than Deaf culture)

- access to and experience of Deaf role models and deaf peers

- school type and academic progress if applicable.

Whether using a sign interpreter or not, the way in which the interviewer communicates with the child is crucial. If the child is using lip-reading, the interviewer must be careful not to exaggerate their lip-patterns or speak overly loudly as this will only distort the lip-patterns making them harder to read, and may make the person appear to be angry or aggressive.

One aspect of the family's functioning that is important to assess is the level of communication between family members. It is not uncommon for the only other person in the family to learn any signs, aside from the deaf child, to be the mother. Even then the mother's signing skills may be very rudimentary, and once the child enters formal education, his or her knowledge of sign language far surpasses anyone else's in the family. This can lead to skewed dynamics within the family, for example when the mother has to 'interpret' what the deaf child says to the rest of the family, or the child can only communicate effectively with his or her parents when a signing teacher is present. Very often parents report no difficulties in communicating with their child, when clearly communication is strained or ineffective and the child may appear to have greater language or communication difficulties than they really do because they have given up trying.

Families referred for behavioural problems in their deaf child(ren) come from diverse ethnic and religious backgrounds. Cultural beliefs about deafness and disability in general will need sensitive exploration, including the family's expectations about the roles that males or females should play within their community. Parents may try to hide their child's deafness from all but the closest family members, or deny that the child has any additional difficulties. They may experience shame or feel blamed, especially when the cause of deafness is genetic or the result of infection that might have been avoided. Alternatively, the religious faith of some parents leads them to believe that a miracle will cure their child's deafness, so they do nothing to intervene in terms of using hearing devices or accessing appropriate educational resources.

Considerable emphasis should be placed on gaining an understanding of the child's social interactions with his or her peers, both hearing and deaf, during the assessment. It is useful to find out who the child's best friends are, whether they sign or not, and the extent to which the child is able to develop close supportive friendships and participate in activities outside school. Opportunities for deaf children to socialize with other hearing-impaired children may be few and far between, as they often have to attend schools that are a long way from their homes and use transport that cannot be tailored to accommodate after-school clubs or activities. In addition, parents do not get the opportunity to meet other parents at the school gates, making it harder for them to foster friendships for their children.

Case example: Out of control

Flora, aged four-and-a-half, was referred to the clinic as a result of concerns from her parents and nursery school teachers, that she was 'uncontrollable' and a danger to her younger brother and other children. Her severe sensori-neural hearing loss had been identified when she was two years old, and consistent hearing-aid use had never been established, due to generalized problems of non-compliance. Flora communicated through gesture, pointing and facial expression and used between eight and ten recognizable spoken words. The pre-school provision she attended employed an aural/oral approach and actively discouraged the use of sign language. Flora threw severe temper tantrums at least twice a day, where she would scream, throw objects and kick or bite others, including her two-year-old brother who was hearing and communicated easily with their parents. Flora frequently covered her face with her hand when someone tried to talk to her, and only gave eye contact on her own terms. Flora's mother believed that the only way to deal with Flora's demands was to let her have whatever she wanted straight away, both in order to avoid a tantrum and because she felt that it was impossible to explain or negotiate with Flora due to her lack of understanding of speech. Flora's father agreed that it was impossible to 'talk' Flora into 'behaving', and therefore would smack her when she disobeyed him, often without warning.

Formulation of behavioural problems and disorders

'Formulation' is a term used primarily by clinical psychologists and is an individualized account of the difficulties that the patient and his or her family faces, encompassing predisposing, precipitating and perpetuating (maintaining) factors. It is the synthesis of the knowledge gained during the assessment process and is based on psychological theory and research to provide a framework for describing a problem, how it developed and is being maintained. A formulation may comprise a number of provisional hypotheses regarding the child and family's difficulties, and provides the basis from which interventions are suggested. A number of different theoretical approaches may inform the formulation, to a large degree depending on the background and preferences of the psychologist involved, for example psychodynamic, cognitive-behavioural, systemic or humanistic approaches. However, an alternative way of looking at a child's difficulties is to consider the biological, psychological and social factors involved – the 'biopsychosocial' model. This can be particularly useful when thinking about the difficulties facing a deaf child, as all three areas usually play a significant part in shaping their development and behaviour.

Case example: Always in trouble

Kieron is a nine-year-old boy referred as a result of difficulties both at home and school. He was born 12 weeks prematurely, and had a moderate hearing loss. His mother, a single parent who was on anti-depressant medication, described Kieron as having a battery that never runs down. He would be constantly fiddling with objects, even whilst apparently engaged in watching TV, and be unable to stick with one task for more than a few minutes. Getting him to do his homework was a constant battle, and his literacy skills were particularly poor, even taking into account his hearing-impairment. He would have frequent angry outbursts, especially towards his three younger siblings. Kieron attended a mainstream school where he was the only child with a hearing-impairment. He had developed no stable friendships, and most of his peer group avoided engaging with him as he was never able to stick with the rules of their games, and could be aggressive at times. His teachers described him as being disruptive and attention-seeking, constantly putting his hand up to ask what they felt were unnecessary questions.

In Figure 2.1 information from Kieron's assessment is presented as one possible formulation of his difficulties. In this simple formulation the predisposing factors are primarily the biological ones, and the psychological and social factors are likely to be contributing to the maintenance of Kieron's difficulties. In this example there is no clear precipitating factor – Kieron's behaviour problems emerged over a period of time, becoming steadily worse during his primary school years. Following the initial assessment it was clear that further information was needed in order to fully understand Kieron's difficulties. In particular, a thorough assessment of his cognitive abilities, language and literacy skills was needed in order to determine his special educational needs more precisely, so that appropriate support could be provided in these areas. Further consideration of his communication and social difficulties was also indicated in order to enable him to improve his peer relationships and join in more at school.

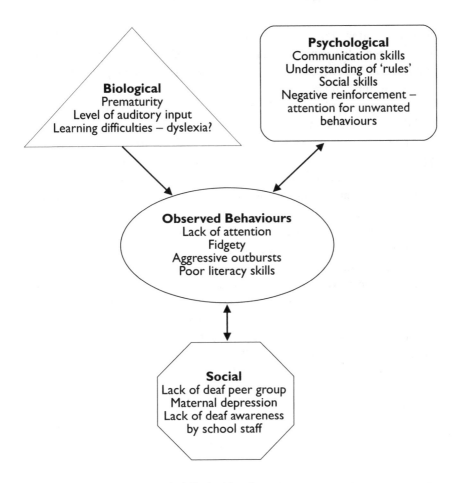

Figure 2.1 Formulation of Kieron's difficulties from his assessment

Intervention

As with the assessment process, intervention should be multi-faceted and multi-professional for hearing-impaired children with behavioural disorders or problems, especially where the difficulties occur in a variety of contexts. In pre-school children, peripatetic teachers of the deaf are in an ideal position to be able to support families and implement intervention strategies, as they are most likely to have regular contact with the child over an extended period of time. Class teachers, special educational needs teachers and school teachers of the deaf are also likely to play a pivotal role where behaviours are impacting on the child's academic progress or social and emotional well-being at school. Thus, there needs to be close and regular liaison between the child mental health team and other agencies such as education and social services. In addition to working in collaboration with these other agencies, the community mental health services, specialist psychological services linked to audiological or cochlear implant services, or specialist Deaf mental health services may offer therapeutic sessions to the child and family.

In common with other fields within mental health, a variety of theoretical and therapeutic models or approaches may be used, depending on the training and preferences of the clinicians involved, and the nature of the presenting problems. The deaf child may be offered individual psychotherapy sessions, cognitive-behavioural therapy or group therapy with other hearing-impaired children. Alternatively all members of the family may be engaged in systemic therapy, or the child's parents may be advised to use behavioural strategies to improve behaviour in a toddler. Clearly, it is not possible to provide detailed information here on all the possible approaches for every type of behaviour problem. Indeed, it is not even necessary, as there are more similarities than differences when a hearing-impaired child is involved. However, as with assessment, it remains absolutely essential that the child's communication abilities and needs are met throughout therapy and that they are fully engaged in the process, dependent on their age and developmental levels. Where the child has severely limited spoken or sign language skills, the use of drawing, sculpting or role play may be necessary. In some cases, work needs to be done with the child before starting the therapeutic intervention 'proper', on the child's 'theory of mind' skills (appreciating that others may have differing beliefs and needs from their own) and their understanding and use of the language of emotions (see Chapter 5 for more information on theory of mind).

Promoting effective communication

We are hoping that it is clear from the above discussions that the fundamental problem facing hearing-impaired children, which makes a major contribution to most if not all of their other difficulties, is their delay in acquiring age-appropriate language and communication skills. In this final section we will outline some of the strategies that can be used to promote effective communication with hearing-impaired children from infancy onwards. Whilst many of them may appear obvious, and do indeed come naturally to some parents and other adults involved with the child, others are less so and may need to be explicitly taught or modelled.

General

Before trying to communicate with a deaf child it is helpful to follow a few basic guidelines to make the communication more effective and less frustrating for both participants. As much as possible reduce distractions such as the television or radio, or if necessary, go into another room where there are no other people or noise. With a young child it is important to get down to their level, so that your face is at roughly the same height as theirs, face them directly and make sure you have gained their attention before you start. Don't eat or cover your mouth in any way when talking, as this distorts lip-patterns, but don't speak too slowly or loudly either, as this can also make it more difficult for the child to follow you. Using lots of facial expressions and gestures to supplement your speech or signs is useful, and it may be necessary to ask the child to repeat back what you have said, to check that they have understood correctly.

Pre-verbal skills
EYE CONTACT
Many hearing-impaired children have poor or fleeting eye contact, or may avoid it altogether. Increasing eye contact allows the child to gain more from social interactions and learn more about language through facial expression, lip-patterns and signs. Games such as peep-po, using masks or sunglasses and holding toys or objects up to your face all encourage the child to look at the person's face. The child can be reinforced for looking at someone's face by only giving them the toy once they have made eye contact.

ATTENTION
Good attention and concentration skills are essential for a child to be able to begin to understand language. Almost any activity that engages a child's interest can be used to extend their attention skills, but activities such as play dough, threading beads, blowing up a balloon, inset puzzles and action rhymes are often useful ones in this context. Ultimately, any activity that is of particular interest to the child will work best.

COPYING
Copying is an important skill as it provides a foundation for developing other skills and for improving observation. Children can be encouraged to copy funny faces and action nursery rhymes such as 'Round and round the garden like a teddy bear', 'Wind the bobbin up' and 'The wheels on the bus'. Older children enjoy 'Simon says' games and can be encouraged to copy pretend play with dolls, cars, farm or zoo animals or everyday activities such as cooking or cleaning.

TURN-TAKING
Most young children find it difficult to wait, share and take turns at some point. The ability to take turns is important for communication in terms of conversation turn-taking and social skills. Develop turn-taking in a one-to-one

situation with a child, before expecting them to cope with waiting for several other children before it is their turn. Keep in control of the activity by holding on to the equipment being used, only handing over one piece at a time, when it is the child's turn. Almost any activity can be turned into an opportunity to develop turn-taking – kicking or throwing a ball, stirring a cake mix, turning the pages of a picture book or lifting the flaps, putting shapes in a shape-sorter or rolling cars towards one another.

PLAY

Play provides endless opportunities for developing language and communication. It takes many forms – exploratory, physical, make-believe and symbolic, all of which can be accompanied by commenting, asking questions and rephrasing the child's attempts at speech or sign. It is important to always take the child's lead and go at the child's pace, resisting the temptation to make the child play in a particular way or try to say specific words, when they may not be ready or capable.

Conclusions

Behaviour problems and disorders are very common amongst hearing-impaired children, irrespective of their mode of communication. They are strongly associated with aetiologies of deafness where there is central nervous system involvement, or additional disabilities caused by infection or as part of a syndrome. Fluent, effective communication between parents and their child during the child's earliest years, whether in spoken or sign language, appears to be crucial in encouraging psychological well-being throughout childhood and beyond. Therefore, one of the most central roles of psychologists and other professionals working with very young hearing-impaired children is to promote the development of positive, effective communication skills as soon as a hearing-impairment is identified. When serious behavioural problems occur, families need access to services with appropriately trained and skilled professionals, which is timely and mindful of the specific needs of hearing-impaired children. Although highly specialist services for the Deaf do exist, they are currently few and far between and therefore considerably over-subscribed. The need for assessment and intervention in the broader hearing-impaired population could be met by community services, with support and input from specialist services when necessary. We would encourage any mental health professional referred a deaf child and his or her family to embrace this challenge and discover the rewards of working with this group of children.

3 Self-concept, Self-esteem and the Development of Identity

'Why am I deaf but my sister can hear?' 'Will I get married to a deaf person?' 'Will my children be like me [i.e. deaf]?' 'Will I be like my family [i.e. able to hear] when I grow up?' These are all questions we have been asked by deaf children who are questioning who they are, why they are different from their family or peers and what this means for their future. The issue of identity is of particular significance to many deaf people as we shall see later on in this chapter. Even when deaf individuals do not identify themselves with the Deaf culture or community, they must still develop an identity that incorporates their deafness. How they achieve this and the extent to which they are comfortable with this identity will have implications for their self-esteem and emotional well-being throughout childhood, adolescence and beyond.

This chapter will consider the various contexts within which deaf children grow up and how these may shape their developing identity. Following a brief account of the theoretical background to identity development we will review the available research literature on the identity and self-esteem of deaf children and adolescents, and the association between them. The remainder of the chapter will focus on clinical work with deaf children where their identity is of significance in the presentation, and the therapeutic work undertaken with them.

Terminology

A variety of terms are used when describing the concept of identity – self-concept, self-image, self-schemas and, of course, the word 'identity' itself. Self-concept, self-image and identity are often used interchangeably and are the sum of the individual's knowledge and understanding of him- or herself, including aspects such as their physical, social and psychological attributes. For example, a person may see him- or herself as tall, attractive, shy, clever, boring, generous, sporty and so on. For the remainder of this chapter we will use the term self-concept to refer to this global view of all aspects of the self. Because the term 'identity' has very particular connotations in the field of deafness, we will use it more specifically to refer to deaf children's perception of themselves in relation to their hearing status.

Self-concept is important in influencing how we behave and relate to others, in turn influencing experiences of success or failure. Of clinical or thera-peutic significance is the fact that self-concept is learned throughout one's life, being shaped and reshaped as a result of experiences and one's perception of those experiences. Emotional problems for the individual are likely to arise if they perceive there to be inconsistencies between their self-concept and experi-ences and these inconsistencies cannot be resolved by altering the self-concept in a way that is acceptable to the individual. The more central a belief is to the person's self-concept the harder it is to change it and the longer it takes to do so. Having said this, the development of self-concept is a continuous process with ongoing assimilation of new ideas and rejection of old ideas, although the self-concept is likely to become more stable during adulthood. Given that the development of self-concept is based on the accumulation of experiences and the individual's interpretation of them from infancy onwards, we might predict that language plays a central role in its formation. It is well established that deaf children lag behind their peers in their understanding and use of vocabulary relating to emotions (e.g. Dyck and Denver 2003; Dyck *et al.* 2004) and this is likely to have an impact on their development of a fully differentiated, multi-faceted self-concept. An awareness of the thoughts, feelings and experi-ences of other people makes it easier for children to understand their own expe-riences and emotions. In deaf children, the language deficits and communica-tion difficulties typically experienced, particularly in early childhood, will affect their awareness of what other people experience and hence their under-standing of their own internal world. However, as yet the impact of language on the development of self-concept is an area that has not been empirically studied in young hearing-impaired children. Indeed, there is very little research evidence on the development of self-concept generally in hearing-impaired children, but what is available will be reviewed below.

The formation of a healthy, positive self-image may pose significant challenges for a child when family, peers, community or societal evaluations of the individual are perceived by the individual as being negative, particularly if inaccurate. If such negative evaluations are experienced on a regular basis and especially if the person making the evaluation is valued or influential, this is likely to result in anxiety, depression or poor self-esteem. On this basis it is easy to conceive how deaf children growing up in an environment where communication is restricted, and where they do not have access to positive Deaf role models, may suffer poor self-esteem or other psychological difficulties.

This brings us to the concept of self-esteem or self-worth, which is closely related to that of self-concept. Self-esteem can be defined as the subjective appraisal of oneself as intrinsically positive or negative to some degree. Self-esteem concerns the attributes we believe we hold and the value we place on them. It can be construed as either 'state' or 'trait', that is, as a temporary psychological position or enduring personality characteristic. It derives from perceptions of competence, mastery and acceptance. Once again, it can be readily hypothesized that deaf children are at increased risk of having poor self-esteem as a result of their experiences of isolation, difficulty communicating, learning to read and write and interacting with hearing peers. Desselle (1994) postulates that poor self-esteem is more likely to be present if the child's parents are not also deaf. She also points out that deafness does not directly cause poor self-esteem, but rather the degree to which the child is able to communicate contributes to the development of self-worth. If parents view deafness as a defect or disability and this is conveyed to the child over time, we might expect negative consequences for the child's development of self-esteem.

Both self-concept and self-esteem are typically measured using self-report questionnaires assessing a variety of domains such as academic achievements, friendships, family relationships, physical appearance and an overall or global evaluation. Whilst a number of measures are available, most are now somewhat outdated and were not developed with hearing-impaired children in mind. A number of questionnaires have been adapted to accommodate the language needs of deaf respondents, for example by presenting the items in sign language or simplifying the written language used. These changes are not always subjected to tests of their validity or reliability and normative data for hearing-impaired children is not usually available for the revised measure. The measures tend to be available only for older children or young adults as the linguistic demands are too great for younger children. Also, they often confound, or at least confuse the ideas of self-concept and self-esteem, making it difficult to interpret findings and compare results across studies.

Thus, in summary, our working definitions are that the self-concept is how a person views him- or herself, the characteristics they attribute to themselves. Self-esteem is how they feel about this perception – the evaluative component that results in an emotional response.

In the field of deafness the term 'identity' needs to be distinguished from that of self-concept, and has very strong, specific connotations. Rather than encompassing the perception of the self across all areas of functioning, Deaf identity refers to an individual's perception of him- or herself as a member of the Deaf community. The phrase 'Deaf cultural identity' is used to describe the position of some deaf people of belonging to a distinct group, which separates them from their hearing counterparts. It is to this issue we now turn.

Deaf culture and Deaf identity

People whose hearing acuity is not within the normal range may be variously described as deaf, hard of hearing or hearing-impaired. All of these are commonly used by members of the medical profession and others who work in this field. However, to many, these words, and particularly 'hearing-impaired', imply a disability or handicap that should be corrected if possible, and may have strongly negative connotations. This medical model of deafness is one that the majority of parents of congenitally deaf and deafened (e.g. by meningitis) children, and deafened adults, find they are thrown into and become caught up in its powerful system. In contrast, the term 'Deaf' with a capital D has come to refer to people who regard themselves as part of the Deaf community or Deaf culture, who view their deafness positively and vehemently refute that it is disabling. Their contention is that it is the society in which they are required to function that produces the handicap, not the deafness per se. Membership of the Deaf community is not a function of the degree of deafness, but more strongly associated with the extent to which the person shares the language, beliefs and values of the Deaf culture. Thus, although the most expected mode of 'entry' to the community is by deaf children of deaf parents from birth onwards, membership is also conferred to deaf individuals who may have become exposed to Deaf culture at various stages in their life, through their educational setting or during adulthood. Given that the majority of deaf children have hearing parents, this group forms a sizeable proportion of the Deaf community. Also, it is not impossible for a hearing person to consider him- or herself a member of the Deaf community, through their use of sign language and close affiliation with the social customs, history, education and traditions of the Deaf community.

Deaf cultural values and traditions, like those of other cultures, are most readily passed from one generation to another through modelling by parents or other family members. Alternatively, deaf children may learn about Deaf culture through attendance at Schools for the Deaf, or through a conscious decision on the part of parents to seek out and join with members of the Deaf community, for example at Deaf clubs. Deaf culture has a rich and colourful folklore tradition that plays an essential role in creating and perpetuating Deaf identity through the transmission of the beliefs and values of the Deaf community. The term 'Deaflore' has been coined to refer to the collective knowledge of the Deaf community, including Deaf humour and jokes, legends, riddles, stories, personal narratives, sign language poetry and the sign language games played by children. It also encompasses sign language taboos and conventions of politeness and socially acceptable behaviour that may differ quite markedly from the norms of hearing society. For example, touching someone to gain their attention and maintaining steady eye-gaze throughout a dialogue may be experienced as intrusive or overbearing by hearing people but are essential parts of communication for deaf individuals.

For more information on Deaf culture see Lane (1990) and Ladd (2002). Interesting discussions of whether Deaf culture is a true culture, comparable with ethnic or religious groups, are provided by Davis (2007) and at www.deafculture.com.

Membership of the Deaf community versus the hearing world could be seen as mutually exclusive, and certainly there is a sense that entry into the Deaf community requires some degree of rejection of the values and attitudes of hearing people. However, development of an individual's identity is a complex process and it is therefore not surprising that many deaf people do not identify with only one culture or group. Glickman and Carey (1993) propose an identity paradigm comprising four possible orientations – culturally hearing, marginal (identifying with neither the hearing nor Deaf worlds), culturally Deaf, and bicultural (equally at home in both Deaf and hearing worlds). A wide variety of factors will affect the extent to which a deaf child develops an identity along these possible lines, including the attitudes of his or her parents towards deafness, the use of sign language in the home and at school, his or her peer relationships and access to Deaf role models.

Theories of identity development

One of the first tasks in the development of an individual identity is to learn to distinguish between the 'self' and 'other'. Infants of around 18 months old are able to recognize themselves in a mirror and point to a picture of themselves when someone says their name. At around the same time they are beginning to develop self-awareness, the capacity to perceive their own attributes, feelings and abilities. This can be seen when the children refer to themselves and their actions, for example by describing what they are doing during play – 'make tea' or 'find book'. This is followed by the ability to describe states such as 'hurt' and 'thirsty', and attributes such as 'clever' and 'good'. In the early childhood years, up to the age of about seven, when children are asked to describe themselves they tend to do so in terms of physical attributes and favourite activities. Over the next few years the emphasis changes such that greater weight is placed on behavioural characteristics, and finally by early adolescence the focus is more on psychological traits, with children defining the self in terms of their inner thoughts and feelings. It is likely that the development of the self-concept starts at an earlier age in children than we think, as in most children the ability to understand language exceeds the ability to make verbal reports for a consider-able period of time. In support of this, Eder (1990) showed that children as young as three years were able to make consistent choices between statements describing personality traits, as applied to themselves. This clearly has implica-tions for our understanding of the early development of self-awareness and self-concept in young deaf children, who are very likely to have impoverished receptive as well as expressive language. The probable consequence of this is delayed development of the self-concept relative to that of their hearing peers, although there is no empirical evidence exploring this issue.

Although formation of identity starts during infancy, the greatest period of consolidation is usually considered to be during the adolescent years. It would not be possible to have a discussion of identity development during adolescence without mentioning the work of Erik Erikson (1968) who proposed a theory of eight stages of psychosocial development, the fifth of which concerns adoles-cence, and is characterized by the conflict between identity and role confusion, with emphasis on peer relationships. Erikson considered identity to be not only about the individual and his or her internal world – how they view themselves – he believed that to achieve a true identity it is also important for there to be consistency between how adolescents conceive themselves to be, and how they perceive others to see them. This requires a level of cognitive ability, and in particular meta-cognitive understanding and 'theory of mind' capability, the development of which is typically delayed in deaf children. So once again, it is likely that the process of forming a coherent, fully developed identity is a greater challenge for deaf children.

Following the work of Erikson, Marcia (1993) focused on the concepts of choice and commitment in identity status, suggesting that the sense of identity is largely determined by the choices we make for or against specific personal and social traits, and the degree of commitment to those choices. He proposed four permutations of choice and commitment: identity confusion, when the person has not (yet) chosen their place in life and has no desire to commit to the (unchosen) roles they do occupy; identity foreclosure when the person has not made many definite role choices but is willing to commit to some values, goals or roles for the future; identity moratorium, which describes the individual who appears 'flighty' – making choices but not committing to them fully; and finally, identity achievement where the person makes their identity choices and commits to them. This paradigm is helpful when thinking about the choices deaf adolescents may be faced with in terms of their identity as a deaf person, and whether they want to embrace Deaf culture and become part of the Deaf community.

Woodward (1997) has argued that a person's identity is defined by difference, inclusion versus exclusion, 'insiders' versus 'outsiders', 'us' or 'them'. Differences in hearing status can readily be construed in terms of such opposites – normally hearing versus deaf/hearing-impaired or hard of hearing, leading to the perception of inclusion or exclusion from the Deaf or hearing worlds.

Finally, the work of Newman and Newman (1976) is relevant to our understanding of identity development in deaf children and adolescents. They explored the importance of membership of a defined peer group in the 13–17-year age group. They proposed that young people use peer groups to gain a sense of self in relation to others in society, where the family unit serves this function in younger children. This broadens the possible range of role models available to the young person and allows them to explore different ways of thinking and behaving without having to commit themselves until ready. One crucial aspect of comparisons with a peer group is the status of that group. Where the group is a minority one, as in the case of deaf people, that group is often perceived by the majority group(s) as being of lower status and may become stigmatized. As a consequence it could be assumed that basing one's identity on comparisons with the minority group would result in psychological problems. This is an issue that will be explored further in the research section below.

Research

In this review of the published literature on self-concept, identity and self-esteem the papers are classified as relating to one of these categories according to the authors' choice of terminology. However, many do not make a clear distinction between the concepts, either using the terms interchangeably or employing measures that are somewhat ambiguous in what they are actually measuring.

Self-concept

Relatively few studies have examined self-concept in hearing-impaired children and adolescents. Early studies such as that of Craig (1965) suggested that deaf children display 'poorer' self-concepts than their hearing peers, even when age, gender, intelligence, degree of hearing loss and parental occupation are taken into account. Cates (1991) examined the self-concept of 68 pre-lingually pro-foundly deaf 8–19-year-olds attending a residential School for the Deaf, compared with that of an equal number of hearing children in the same age range. The children completed the Piers-Harris Children's Self-concept Scale (Piers 1984) and their teachers rated them using the Behavioural Academic Self-esteem Scale (Coopersmith and Gilberts 1982). Cates found no differences in overall self-concept between the groups, whether rated by the individuals themselves or their teachers. However, he did find that the perceptions of the teachers of the deaf children (who were themselves, almost without exception, hearing), were not very closely in line with the children's own self-perceptions.

As we noted earlier, the self-concept of young deaf children has received almost no attention, most probably because of the difficulties assessing self-concept when language skills are very poorly developed. However, Culross (1985) provides an exception in her study of 255 hearing-impaired children aged five to eight years attending a variety of school settings. She used the Picto-rial Self-concept Scale (Bolea, Felker and Barnes 1971) and found it to have good reliability and adequate validity in this group. Unfortunately we have been unable to find any further reference to the use of this measure in the literature, for example comparing hearing with deaf children, or deaf children with deaf parents with deaf children of hearing parents, and so on.

One of the factors frequently hypothesized to be influential in determining the self-concept of deaf children is their school setting, in particular the extent to which they are educated with other deaf children. Where they are isolated from deaf peers, and therefore it is assumed that they will compare themselves with their hearing peers, it is usually predicted that self-concept will suffer. The importance of social comparison, in other words the influence of comparisons with others on children's self-concept has been emphasized by Harter (1986). She found that academic self-concept scores were related to the comparison group adopted by learning-disabled and developmentally disabled children. Van Gurp (2001) examined this issue explicitly in secondary-school-age deaf children using a self-report measure that had been modified linguistically and validated for deaf students. The questionnaire had scales assessing appearance, parental relations, peer relations, reading, maths, general school and general self. Results suggested that children in 'units' or 'resource' provision (i.e. educated part of the time just with other deaf children, but in the mainstream classroom for the remainder of lessons) have better overall self-concept scores and scores relating to perception of maths ability. Within the group of children attending units, there was no difference in self-concept between those who used predominantly manual methods of communication and those who were predominantly oral. However, the results are difficult to interpret as there are no consistent patterns relating to the degree of integration with hearing peers and for which academic subjects.

As in so many aspects of the development of deaf children, communication competence appears to be of importance in the development of self-concept. Silvestre, Ramspott and Pareto (2006) assessed conversational skills and self-concept in the context of different school settings. Their sample included 56 moderately to profoundly deaf 6–18-year-olds who all had hearing parents. The children attended integrated schools using oral communication methods. The authors report a significant relationship between a positive self-concept and conversational competence, suggesting that conversational skills could be one area usefully targeted for explicit teaching amongst deaf children.

Whilst these studies provide interesting insights into some aspects of deaf children's self-concept, they all have one significant drawback in terms of their validity – the dimensions of self-concept are those considered relevant by the researchers (or more specifically by those who developed the questionnaires) and not the individuals themselves. It is possible that some of the attributes on which the children are asked to rate themselves are not those that they consider personally applicable or of importance, and other more relevant attributes are not included. However, there is one approach to the study of self-concept that overcomes this – Personal Construct and Repertory Grid methodology. This is based on the work of Kelly (1955) who argued that through one's interpretation of events and experiences we build up a set of explanatory theories, a process that leads to the formation of 'constructs', which influence how we view ourselves and others and how we interact with the world. Constructs include attributes such as friendly, shy, generous and lonely, and exist on continua, which may differ from one person to another. For example, a construct for one person may be friendly-shy, but for another it may be friendly-unsociable, which has subtly different meanings. This theoretical approach led to a method of assessing personal constructs, called Repertory Grids (Fransella, Bell and Banister 2004) in which the individual generates a number of constructs based on comparisons between 'elements', or people, either specific people they know (my best friend, my brother/sister) or a generalized person (someone I like, a teacher). Once the constructs have been established, each of the elements are rated on those constructs, producing the Repertory Grid. Grids also often include the elements 'myself' and 'my ideal self' or 'myself as I would like to be' as the discrepancy between these can provide a measure of self-esteem, in addition to a more general self-concept.

Given the potential for this approach to inform us regarding the self-perceptions of deaf individuals it is disappointing that so few studies have capitalized on it. However, there are two relevant studies separated by a span of more than 25 years. The first, by Ballantine (1981) examined the constructs of 27 adolescents aged 16–20 years who were still attending school and were pre-lingually moderately to profoundly deaf. The Repertory Grids produced by the students were analysed to examine how the students construed themselves and to produce a measure of the extent to which they defined themselves as being like other deaf people. Two main findings emerged. First, 11 of the 13 most commonly elicited constructs used to describe themselves were rated as positive (by independent judges), for example friendly, intelligent, not angry, happy and confident. In contrast, of the 13 most commonly elicited constructs describing 'a deaf individual', eight were rated as negative (e.g. unhappy, unenthusiastic, angry, unintelligent, unhelpful), two as neutral (unlike self and like self) and only three as positive (friendly, happy and not worried). This indicates that although the students described themselves in very positive terms, their view of the attributes of deaf people generally was much more negative. Ballantine also used the grids to explore the degree of acceptance of deafness amongst the students and concluded that there was a high degree of denial of their deafness, because the students identified strongly with neither deaf nor hearing people.

The only other study to use Repertory Grid methodology in an exploratory manner is that of Mance and Edwards (in preparation) who focused on a younger group of adolescents aged 12–18 years, who were cochlear implant users. They were concerned with understanding the relationship between self-concept and psychological well-being (anxiety, depression, self-esteem) in view of the suggestion that cochlear implants may leave deaf children (and later adults) 'culturally homeless', neither part of the Deaf nor hearing worlds. Results suggested that identifying with a hearing peer group was associated with higher levels of psychological well-being, but identifying with a deaf peer group was not. This can be accounted for if we assume that those children who receive cochlear implants are exposed to strongly pro-hearing, oral role models and expectations, and that this influences their desired comparison group. As anticipated, it was also found that the closer the individual perceived themselves now to be to their ideal or future self, the higher their level of psychological well-being.

Overall, these studies of self-concept in deaf children and adolescents have provided inconsistent findings in terms of how deaf children view themselves. Even if negative self-concept is only an issue for a proportion of deaf children, it is essential that this aspect of their development is not ignored or underestimated, as it is clear that there are consequences for future psychological well-being.

Self-esteem

A greater, although still small, number of studies have examined the self-esteem of deaf children or adults, but again with mixed findings. Bat-Chava (1993) carried out a meta-analysis of the studies available at that time, the majority (87%) of which were unpublished master's or doctoral theses. Results suggested the communication mode used in the classroom was not related to self-esteem but that use of sign language rather than oral communication by parents was associated with higher self-esteem. Those studies that examined parental hearing status as a variable (of which there were 12) indicated a significant positive effect on self-esteem of having deaf parents. This was explored further by Crowe (2003) who, unlike in previous research, found that amongst deaf college students, those who had two deaf parents had higher self-esteem scores than those who had two hearing parents or one deaf and one hearing parent, *regardless of use of sign by the parents*. A possible explanation for this finding is linked to the degree to which parents belong to the Deaf community and are able to convey the positive attitudes towards deafness, and the cultural perspective of deafness, to their children. Also the high status of 'native' members of the Deaf culture (i.e. where this has been passed on from parents to children through family lineage), is likely to have a positive influence on the self-esteem of their children.

A number of more recent studies have sought to determine what factors are important in influencing the self-esteem of deaf children. For example, Woolfe (2001) examined the role of deaf versus hearing siblings in determining self-esteem in deaf children aged 10–14 years, but found no significant effect of sibling hearing status. However, there was a significant main effect of parental hearing status such that those children with deaf parents had higher self-esteem than those with hearing parents. Woolfe concluded that the hearing status of the parents is the more powerful influence on self-esteem, possibly because of their more powerful status and the significant role they play in making choices for their deaf child and the need for effective communication with the child regarding all aspects of the child's life.

Jambor and Elliott (2005) also looked at the contribution of communication in the home to deaf young adults' self-esteem but did not find a significant relationship between them. They argue that membership of a minority group such as the Deaf community, despite often being of lower status in society, may protect self-esteem as it enables the individual to disregard the opinions of 'outsiders' to the group, and place greater value on the opinions and appraisals of members of the group. There is also evidence that members of ethnic minority groups who have a strongly integrated, cohesive family background have higher self-esteem (e.g. Way and Robinson 2003). Consistent with this view, Jambor and Elliott's results indicated that identification with culturally Deaf people was positively related to self-esteem. Interestingly they also found that the participants in the study who were able to function well in both the hearing and Deaf worlds tended to have higher self-esteem. They found no effect of the type of school setting attended before college but a trend towards those with a greater degree of hearing loss having higher self-esteem.

Most recently, one study has explored self-esteem in deaf adolescents with cochlear implants. Given the controversy over the use of implants in deaf children, and the potentially negative consequences for self-esteem suggested by some writers (e.g. Evans 1989), this is an important area to investigate. Sahli and Belgin (2006) compared scores on the Rosenberg self-esteem scale (Rosenberg 1965) in a group of 30 12–19-year-olds before and after receiving a cochlear implant, and with a group of similarly aged hearing adolescents. They found no difference between the control group and the deaf adolescents after implantation in their level of self-esteem, but did find that before implantation the deaf children had poorer self-esteem compared with the hearing controls, indicating an increase in self-esteem following implantation. Whether this is directly attributable to the implant is a matter for conjecture.

Whilst there are some conflicting, and some unexpected findings in the literature on self-esteem in deaf children, it does appear that certain factors are influential in enhancing self-esteem in these children. In general, attention has focused on environmental factors such as parenting, the child's social environment, communication in the home and type of schooling as potential contributors to self-esteem, with some significant findings. However, the role of other variables has not been systematically explored, for example genetic factors, intelligence or the presence of medical or physical disorders in addition to the deafness, so the picture is far from complete. In addition, most of the studies were conducted in North America so the applicability of the results to other groups of deaf children must be questioned. Finally, we have tried to focus on deaf children and adolescents, rather than adults, but this restricts the available literature greatly, and a number of studies have been included that focus on older adolescents and young adults. Of course children grow up to become adults, and therefore the results of these studies are of relevance, particularly where they identify factors present during childhood that are associated with positive self-esteem. This can inform our understanding of, and work with, deaf children and adolescents requiring psychological support for problems with achieving a positive self-image and sense of self-worth.

Deaf identity

In this section we will look at those studies that have explicitly explored the development of identity in relation to Deaf culture. Very few published studies look at factors that may influence the development of a Deaf, hearing, bi-cultural or marginal identity (Glickman and Carey 1993). One such study investigates Deaf identity in adults rather than children, but is nonetheless of relevance to us in that the authors ask the participants to reflect on their experiences during childhood and adolescence. Nikolaraizi and Hadjikakou (2006) used qualitative research methods to explore the role of school on the Deaf identity development of 25 adults educated within the Greek system of special Schools for the Deaf, units for deaf children within 'general' schools or general schools with no additional provision. Analysis of the interview transcripts led to the participants being categorized as having hearing, Deaf or bi-cultural identities. None of the participants were considered to have a marginal identity. All seven of the participants with a hearing identity had attended general schools, three of which had units attached to them. This was not typically viewed positively by the participants, particularly at secondary school level; communication was experienced as very difficult, as was understanding the lessons, and feelings of low acceptance by their peers were common. This group had predominantly hearing friends and used oral language to communicate, although some also used sign language when necessary. In contrast, those participants who were considered to have a Deaf identity had spent most of their school years in Schools for the Deaf. Although their academic experiences were mixed, these participants reflected on the positive impact of being able to communicate easily with their peers in sign language. These deaf adults expressed feeling most comfortable with other deaf people and preferred to communicate in sign. The last group, those with a bicultural identity, had attended either general schools or both general and Schools for the Deaf. They explicitly considered themselves to be part of both the hearing and Deaf worlds, but also described balancing the two as being difficult, and communicating in sign language was generally preferred. The social context served to define whether they feel deaf or Deaf at any particular time.

Israelite, Ower and Goldstein (2002) focus on identity development in 'hard of hearing' (HH) adolescents where HH encompasses all levels of hearing loss including severe or profound loss, and communication is primarily through audition and speech. HH people do not identify themselves as a minority group in the way members of the culturally Deaf community do, are diverse in terms of the impact of their hearing loss on communication, education, work and social experiences, and have an identity that contrasts with that of the identity of culturally Deaf people. Israelite and colleagues interviewed seven adolescents aged 14–17 years who had previously been educated through a combination of segregated classes and partial mainstreaming. They used qualitative methodology to identify common themes or categories of response. Each participant also completed written questionnaires about their views on the educational and social consequences of being HH. Results indicated that this group of adolescents generally defined themselves in relation to hearing people, but in terms of different abilities to perceive sound rather than as intrinsically different people. In contrast, they also tended to see themselves as distinct from culturally Deaf people, valuing being able to communicate and integrate with hearing people in a way that they perceived culturally Deaf people to be unable to do. They emphasized wanting to 'fit in' with their hearing peers at school and be accepted by both their peers and teachers, but feeling marginalized, 'outsiders'. The authors conclude that HH adolescents do form a group that is different from both hearing and Deaf groups, with distinct identities, supporting Woodward's (1997) contention that identity develops through perception of difference. Israelite et al. (2002) stress the crucial role of teachers in promoting participation, self-acceptance and a sense of belonging, in order to foster feelings of social competence and confidence.

These studies suggest that the educational experiences of deaf children play an important role in moulding their identity, in addition to the influence of the family. The implications of choices made by deaf children, especially during the adolescent years, should not be underestimated as they will shape the individual's future social and emotional functioning, and therefore psychological well-being.

Clinical presentations of identity or self-esteem problems in deaf children

More often than not a deaf child who has been referred for psychological assessment, whose primary psychological needs are around their identity or self-esteem, will not have previously been considered to have problems in these areas. Depending on the age of the child, their presentation, or the problems identified by adults around them, may be quite different.

Behaviour (externalizing) problems

A younger child (i.e. primary-school-aged) may be described as having behaviour problems, for example being disobedient or defiant at home, fighting with siblings, unusually angry, or disruptive in the classroom. In the family environment, conflict with brothers and sisters is sometimes the result of the deaf child making unfavourable comparisons with them, or feeling left out or neglected by family members who cannot communicate freely with them. Children may choose not to conform to the expectations of their parents as a way of asserting their independence and making themselves feel as if they 'count' within the family system. Whilst this strategy may have the desired effect at one level, insofar as the child will gain attention from it, in the longer term it is likely to lead to poorer self-esteem as the child receives negative feedback from others about his or her behaviour. Deaf children who are having difficulty incorporating their hearing loss into their identity in a positive way may try to develop an alternative identity that distinguishes them from their peers or siblings, through engaging in behaviours that set them apart from others. School children who feel as if they don't belong, who are excluded or ridiculed by their peers, but are unable to express themselves effectively to the teachers or other staff, may 'act out', becoming disruptive, inattentive or oppositional.

Internalizing problems

In contrast to these presentations, where the child is exhibiting 'externalizing' behaviour problems, other children, and particularly girls, may present with 'internalizing' problems such as anxiety, low mood and withdrawal. These sorts of difficulties are usually more evident in the school setting, and it is not uncommon for parents to say that their child is angry or difficult to manage at home, but for their teachers to describe them as a model pupil in school. Some children may be described by their teachers as excessively shy, having difficulty making friends amongst either their deaf or hearing peers, or as being a 'loner'. Such children may look sad, cry easily or appear unusually wary of unfamiliar adults or children.

Bullying

Sometimes children are referred for help with dealing with being bullied, a common, but underestimated problem for deaf children. Bullying can take many forms, and is often subtle, and deaf children who cannot communicate effectively are an obvious, easy target. Unfortunately some deaf children deny being bullied when in fact they are, perhaps because they do not fully understand what constitutes bullying, or because they feel embarrassed or do not want to have another reason for being different from other children. Being teased or bullied is obviously likely to impact on self-esteem but it may also lead to the child questioning why they are being singled out in this way, why they are different from their peers. The situation can be particularly confusing and distressing if the bully is another deaf child.

Academic difficulties

Another group of children where the underlying issues may be related to identity or self-esteem are those who appear to have academic difficulties. Such children may be referred because they are not making the progress expected in learning to read or write, or develop mathematical skills. They are often described as having poor attention and concentration skills, memory problems or lacking motivation to learn. Parents may also say that their child refuses to comply with homework and seems to forget even the simplest things they have been taught. Occasionally the situation becomes so bad that school refusal is the trigger for a request for psychological help.

Adolescents

In older children the presentation is often very different, and issues of identity may be explicitly referred to in the request for help. Any of the problems described above may still be present, but during the adolescent years deaf children are more likely to articulate their thoughts and feelings about being deaf, either with their parents, a trusted teacher or perhaps school counsellor. Help is usually only sought when such discussions are accompanied by anxiety or distress in the young person, or their parents feel unable to provide them with adequate answers, perhaps because of their own feelings about their child's deafness and the choices they would like their child to make. Some families seek professional advice as they believe their child may feel more comfortable talking to someone outside the family whose feelings won't be hurt and who can take an impartial, balanced view.

Assessment and formulation

Given the wide variety of possible presentations of difficulties relating to self-esteem or identity, it is essential that a careful, thorough history is taken. This should be from a number of sources, including the child, their family and, with permission, their teachers. This is important because it is not unusual to find very different views on what the problems are, and ideas about the causes of difficulties, from different people. Assessment may need to take place over a number of sessions, and with older children and adolescents it is helpful to spend some time with them on their own (or just with a sign language interpreter if necessary), as many young people feel inhibited talking in front of family members, for fear of upsetting them, shocking them or making them angry.

A considerable amount of background information about the child's hearing loss and its impact should be sought, including:

- the degree of hearing loss

- the aetiology of deafness if known

- age at diagnosis

- communication methods used in the home

- early development

- opportunities for socializing outside the home

- attitudes towards the use of hearing devices such as hearing aids or cochlear implants.

It is also important to gain a full understanding of the family context in terms of deafness. Are there any other members of the immediate or more distant family who are deaf, and how do they communicate? Do the child's parents see deafness as a disability or deficit that needs 'curing', or do they see it as one of the many things that makes their child who they are, and unique? Do they feel that bringing up their deaf child is different from raising their other children, or do they feel they can treat all their children equally in terms of discipline or expectations for achievement?

As with any psychological assessment, a clear picture of the presenting problems needs to be obtained, including the onset, course and maintenance of the problem. One of the primary tasks of assessment is to understand the contribution of all the possible aetiological influences, such as genetic predisposition, learning and modelling or individual temperament. For example, it may be necessary to distinguish between externalizing problems that are due to parenting practices and those that are the result of persistent exclusion from a peer group and hence feelings of rejection and inadequacy. Alternatively, it may be necessary to rule out certain diagnoses, as in the case of a child who is restless and distractible in school, whose school work has deteriorated and who seems to be having difficulty concentrating, who may therefore initially appear to have an attention deficit disorder. Different interventions will be appropriate depending on the cause of the child's difficulties, so accurate assessment is essential.

Clearly, some of the most essential information can only be gained from the individuals themselves. This is often easier said than done, as many deaf children do not have the linguistic skills, either orally or in sign, to express themselves as fully as their hearing peers can. However, slow, careful, sensitive questioning, along with the use of media such as modelling clay, pencils or paint if necessary, can reveal the true nature of the child's difficulties. Areas to explore directly with the child might include the following:

- Who communicates most with whom in the family?

- What communication methods do different family members use?

- Is sign language encouraged or discouraged at home?

- What strategies do family members use if there is a breakdown in communication?

- Who understands the child's communication best?

- Who does the child feel most close to emotionally?

- Who would the deaf child choose to talk to if he or she had a problem?

In terms of the wider family context, it is helpful to get an idea of the opportunities the child has for socializing with friends, not linked to school. The child might be asked about whether they have friends who are hearing or deaf, or a mixture of both, and whether they attend a Deaf club or activities run by organizations such as the Deaf Children's Society.

Issues around achievements and relationships at school also need careful exploration. The child should be asked about his or her likes and dislikes at school, favourite subjects and any particular interests or strengths. Their perception of their own abilities in relation to their peers' provides useful information regarding self-concept and self-esteem, as does the perception of their ability to make friends. It is essential to find out about the available peer group for the deaf child – whether they are the only deaf child in the school, the only one in their class, or perhaps the only girl amongst a small number of deaf boys. Alternatively, do they attend a School for the Deaf during the week where they can communicate easily, but have difficulty on returning home at weekends? Are there any deaf teachers or members of staff at their school who can act as role models or advocates for the child? Another area to ask the deaf child about is their use of hearing aids, cochlear implants or other technology within the classroom, and their feelings about this.

Finally, assessment of a deaf child whose difficulties include poor self-esteem or uncertainty over their identity must also include gaining an understanding of any difficulties or disabilities they have in addition to their deafness. In particular, learning difficulties and social communication difficulties (autistic spectrum disorders) are likely to have a significant impact on the child's view of him- or herself and on their interaction with both hearing and deaf peers, and adults. Where, for example, the child has problems with the pragmatic aspects of language or with understanding social rules or conventions, this is likely to lead to poor peer relationships, rejection and isolation, and hence fewer opportunities to explore different identities and develop a positive self-image.

Discussion of the problems that the family or school has requested help with can be supplemented with judicious use of questionnaires, where the language skills of the child make it possible to administer them. A number of standardized measures are available that can provide useful information. One example that we have found deaf children to be able to complete, with some clarification of vocabulary if necessary, is the Beck Youth Inventories – Second Edition for Children and Adolescents (Beck *et al.* 2005). This comprises five scales that can be used separately or in combination, assessing anxiety, depression, anger, disruptive behaviour and self-concept. Whilst they can be used to determine clinical 'caseness' (i.e. the presence of a clinically significant problem), we have found them more useful as a tool for opening a dialogue with the child about his or her thoughts and feelings, and as a pre- and post-intervention outcome measure. However, as with all standardized measures applied to deaf children, considerable caution needs to be exercised when interpreting the results as there is no normative data for deaf children and adolescents.

Having completed the assessment (although it can be argued that assessment is a process that continues throughout the period of therapeutic involvement with the child and family), a formulation of their difficulties should be proposed and shared with the child and family. The formulation should aim to clarify which factors have been instrumental in shaping the child's development of identity, and why problems in this area or with poor self-esteem have arisen. It is likely that this will initially be a very tentative suggestion, and further information may need to be sought and the formulation revised. For example, formal assessment of the child's language skills, specific learning difficulties or specialist assessment of mental health problems may be necessary.

Case example: Frustrated and angry

Chloë is a ten-year-old girl who was deafened by meningitis at the age of 18 months. Her family experienced great difficulty coming to terms with her loss of hearing, and refused to engage with audiological services for the first three years after her illness. She attended a mainstream nursery placement with support from a peripatetic teacher of the deaf, where she had difficulty settling and was described by the teachers as wilful and disruptive. At that point they heard about cochlear implantation and became focused on this as a 'cure' for Chloë's deafness. Despite being advised that an implant might have limited impact on her development of spoken language skills, Chloë's parents decided to go ahead with the procedure. Chloë was given no preparation for the procedure as her language skills were very limited and her parents felt that it would be too difficult for her to understand and therefore would upset her. She continued to attend a mainstream primary school, but it soon became apparent that she was unable to access the curriculum, so was transferred to a school with a 'hearing-impaired unit', one hour's journey from her home. There she started to learn some sign language, but remained considerably delayed in her development of language and communication compared with both her hearing and deaf peers. Chloë's parents remained reluctant to use sign language with her, and her skills soon surpassed theirs. At this point Chloë's teachers, with her parents' permission, requested psychological input, as Chloë was becoming increasingly frustrated and angry and was refusing to wear her cochlear implant, although she acknowledged that she could hear better with it. Her academic progress was also causing great concern. Her parents agreed to the referral primarily because they wanted advice on appropriate secondary school placement.

Intervention

Therapeutic work with children where there are issues of identity and/or self-esteem can take many forms, and may require a flexible, multi-agency approach. Effective intervention may involve sessions with the child alone, group work with other deaf children, group work with hearing peers in the school setting or family therapy. Sometimes the child's needs are best met by working with him or her directly, but in many circumstances it is more helpful for the psychologist to take a more consultative role, perhaps initially assessing the child and family in a clinic context, then working closely with teachers or other community professionals who can provide an ongoing consistent, accessible and flexible service to them. This is especially constructive when the family live a long way from the available specialist deaf mental health services, and attendance at them is experienced as stigmatizing or alienating.

A number of strategies can be used by parents and teachers to promote self-esteem, self-confidence and self-acceptance in deaf children, both as preventative measures and therapeutic ones when problems have been identified. Perhaps the most fundamental one is to allow the child to speak for him- or herself however limited their language skills, not to hurry them and not to try and guess what they want to say, finishing sentences off for them. Adults need to exercise great patience and restraint to do this but the rewards are that the child will feel understood and that their thoughts, needs and opinions are validated.

From an early age, deaf children need to be taught social skills that hearing children learn through experience. For example, deaf children are likely to need to have lots of practice at initiating interactions with other children in order to build friendships. They will need to be given help practising what to say when they meet new children for the first time and when they want to join in games or social activities. Role play is one of the most effective ways of learning these skills, but care must be taken if it is done in a group setting at school, that the deaf child is not singled out as having a 'problem', or open to being patronized by their more articulate peers. Both parents and teachers should emphasize the child's strengths and encourage the child to develop hobbies or special interests, or join clubs. Deaf children can participate in drama, music lessons, dance and sports, as well as learn cookery, art or photography, and these activities can serve the dual purpose of exposing deaf children to social situations where they can make friends, as well as experience a feeling of success and pride in their achievements. As with any child though, attempts and efforts at academic, social or other activities should be acknowledged, rather than success alone. Praise should not be conditional on success or the outcome of efforts but on participation and rising to a challenge.

Deaf children are often surprisingly uninformed about deafness and their own hearing loss in particular. Depending on the child's cognitive and language skills, they can be given information about the cause of their deafness, how the ear works normally and how theirs are different, why they have hearing aids or a cochlear implant and how these work. If they are the only child in their class or school who uses such technology they can be helped to explain it to their classmates, so that they feel empowered rather than isolated or stigmatized. When giving information it is important to do so in small 'chunks' and to check that the child has understood before moving on. Plenty of time must be allowed for the child to digest the information and ask questions and this is likely to take much longer than in hearing children.

Self-esteem and self-worth will also be fostered if deaf children are encouraged not to feel embarrassed about their hearing aids, cochlear implant or other devices, and not to hide them. These need to be a part of everyday life, for example part of the routine of getting dressed in the morning, but not covered by clothing such as scarves or hair bands. Most aids are now available in a variety of colours and fashionable designs and children can be encouraged to choose one they like or that makes a statement about their personality or interests.

In addition to these general strategies for improving self-esteem it is sometimes necessary to work more directly with the child and his or her family. A number of approaches can be helpful, including work with the child, family-based interventions such as Solution-Focused Therapy (see Berg and

Steiner 2003 for a useful introductory text that includes plenty of practical suggestions and case examples) or group work (e.g. the PATHS® curriculum; Greenberg and Kusché 1998) either in a clinic or school setting. As we saw earlier in this chapter, problems with self-esteem or identity are often associated with other emotional, behavioural or learning problems and therefore these may need to be the primary focus of the therapeutic intervention, at least initially.

Cognitive-behavioural therapy (CBT)

With younger school-aged children, allowing them to express their thoughts and feelings about themselves and their deafness may be a new experience and have a positive impact on their mood and self-esteem. However, because of their language deficits, using CBT, even when tailored to the needs and development of children, may be beyond most primary-school-aged deaf children. CBT is about understanding how events and experiences are interpreted and identifying and changing the distortions that occur in cognitive processes. The theoretical basis of CBT proposes that early experiences and parenting lead to the formation of fairly rigid ways of thinking (known as core beliefs or schemas). New information from events is compared with these core beliefs. Information that is perceived as consistent with them is 'filtered' out and reinforces and maintains these beliefs, however unhelpful they may be to the individual's psychological well-being. Everyone experiences a stream of automatic thoughts, some of which are related to our core beliefs, and may be about our view of ourselves, our performance and our future. These thoughts lead to emotional, behavioural and somatic changes, which may be experienced as 'symptoms'. Problems arise when these thoughts (cognitions) are distorted in some way and result in feelings and behaviours that are unwanted or unhelpful.

Therapy involves monitoring thoughts to identify core beliefs, negative automatic thoughts and dysfunctional assumptions, and identifying cognitive distortions. The young person may be encouraged to test out their assumptions through behavioural 'experiments', and also to use strategies such as goal planning, relaxation, anger management and social skills training. They are helped to recognize physical symptoms and emotional responses to situations, and to understand the link between their thoughts, feelings and behavioural responses.

CBT requires the child to be aware of their emotions and able to put them into words, and also be able to access and communicate their thoughts. Therefore, the approach is more likely to be realistic for older deaf children and adolescents. Helping them to access and describe their thoughts and feelings can be facilitated by the use of metaphors, role play and imagery. It may be necessary to work with them on their emotional literacy skills before embarking on the main therapeutic work. A wide variety of helpful strategies and worksheets for working with children within a CBT framework are provided by Stallard (2002), and many of these are appropriate for, or can easily be adapted to, the linguistic needs of deaf young people.

Case example: Not hearing but not deaf

Mary is a 15-year-old deaf girl who was referred for help with severe anxiety relating to school, in particular her inability to speak out in class in front of her classmates without blushing, hyperventilating and feeling nauseous. She attends a mainstream school with specialist provision for hearing-impaired children, of which there are three in her year group. Her parents are both Deaf and BSL is used in the home. However, the approach used at school is aural/oral, and signing is strongly discouraged. Mary has experienced some teasing because her speech intelligibility is poor. She is academically able, but her achievements at school are significantly behind her peers, and she is aware that this will have an impact on her choices for future study and work.

Working with Mary within a CBT framework revealed a number of core beliefs including 'Being deaf is not as good as hearing', 'Believing this means I am betraying my parents', 'I will never get a good job' and 'I am not Deaf because I use speech with some of my friends'. She also identified automatic thoughts such as 'If I speak in class everyone will laugh', 'No one will understand what I am saying' and 'I will fail my exams'. Having learnt to identify these negative automatic thoughts and core beliefs Mary responded well to a combination of challenging and modifying her negative thoughts, relaxation exercises and 'experiments' to test out her beliefs in the classroom. She also spent some time exploring her ideas about her future as a Deaf or deaf person, and with the support of the therapist in sessions for the whole family, discovered what her parents' true attitudes were towards her and her use of speech.

Conclusions

The issue of identity, both personal and cultural, is of such fundamental importance to our understanding of deaf children, that we have considered it in some depth. However, as with all topics in this volume, it would not be difficult to devote an entire book to the subject. Indeed, it has not been possible to consider some aspects of identity in relation to deafness: many deaf children need to develop not only a self-concept that incorporates their deafness, but also one that includes an ethnic or religious identity. They may need to learn more than one spoken language alongside sign language, and accommodate beliefs about deafness or disability from within their family or community that conflict with those of their friends, school teachers or significant others in their lives.

Needless to say, there is currently no empirical research that explores the psychological well-being of children in these complex circumstances.

Whilst there is much still to understand about how deafness influences self-esteem and how the factors that feed into the development of self-esteem interact, we do know that some deaf children struggle with this process. We must constantly be mindful of the possible role of identity issues in deaf children presenting with a range of psychological difficulties of which low self-esteem is only one.

4 Specific Learning Difficulties

In some respects the majority of deaf children do not differ from their hearing counterparts. Despite the language delay experienced by many of them, their general development typically follows a normal trajectory, for example in terms of their gross and fine motor skills, visual perception, reasoning abilities and daily living skills. As a result of the language delay the acquisition of literacy and numeracy skills in deaf children usually lags significantly behind that of their peers. However, all too frequently poor academic progress is attributed solely to the child's hearing-impairment, and the possibility of specific additional learning difficulties is not considered or is left until the child is older, and remedial input is then less effective. Part of the problem also lies in the difficulty diagnosing specific learning difficulties (SLDs) where there is a significant hearing-impairment and this may deter some professionals from pursuing the issue.

Those children for whom deafness is part of a constellation of difficulties (usually of syndromic aetiology), which may include other sensory, medical, motor or learning disabilities, are not the focus of this chapter. Their difficulties are often, but not invariably, more severe and global, and any generalized learning difficulties would 'trump' a specific learning disability in terms of differential diagnosis. However, at the other end of the spectrum, where the child's hearing-impairment may appear to be the only disability, subtle, specific learning difficulties can exist, but go unrecognized and undiagnosed. Hearing-impaired children are not immune to the specific learning difficulties many hearing children experience, which can have such a profound impact on their academic achievement, behaviour and social skills.

In this chapter we will attempt to demonstrate that it is possible to assess hearing-impaired children with a view to diagnosing specific learning difficulties, although we would always acknowledge the need for caution in interpreting assessment results in hearing-impaired children and the importance of recognizing that it may not be possible to adhere rigidly to the diagnostic criteria that are applicable to hearing children. The chapter will focus on three diagnoses – dyslexia, dyspraxia and auditory processing disorder. It should be borne in mind throughout the chapter that we are not referring to deaf children whose only mode of communication is sign language; children need to have a certain degree of oral receptive and expressive language to be able to undergo the assessments needed for these diagnoses.

Definitions of specific learning difficulties

As with many complex topics where defining even the main constructs is contentious, defining each of the types of specific learning difficulty is not straightforward. The task is made more difficult given the overlap in 'symptoms' or presentations of some SLDs. However, for pragmatic purposes, working definitions of SLDs are useful. We have chosen the following definitions of the three disorders to be discussed in this chapter, based on their face validity, clarity and utility in guiding assessment.

Dyslexia

Dyslexia is a neurologically based, often familial, disorder which interferes with the acquisition and processing of language. Varying in degrees of severity, it is manifested by difficulties in receptive and expressive language, including phonological processing, in reading, writing, spelling, handwriting and sometimes arithmetic. (International Dyslexia Association 2002)

Dyspraxia

Dyspraxia is an impairment or immaturity of the organization of movement. It is an immaturity of the way the brain processes information, resulting in messages not being fully transmitted to the body. (Dyspraxia Foundation n.d.)

A disorder of the higher cortical processes involved in the planning and execution of learned, volitional, purposeful movements in the presence of normal reflexes, power, tone, coordination and sensation. (Miller 1986, p.83)

Ideational dyspraxia – difficulty with planning a sequence of coordinated movements.

Ideo-motor dyspraxia – difficulty with executing a plan, even though the plan is known.

Verbal/Oro-motor dyspraxia – difficulty coordinating the movements required to produce speech; difficulty sequencing sounds within a word and forming words into sentences.

Auditory processing disorder (APD)

There are several useful definitions of AP and APD of varying levels of specificity:

APD is a deficit in the processing of information received that is specific to the auditory modality that may be exacerbated in unfavourable acoustic environments and may be associated with difficulties in listening, speech understanding, language development and learning. (Jerger and Musiek 2000, pp.467–474)

Difficulties in the processing of auditory information in the central nervous system demonstrated by poor performance in one or more of sound localization and lateralization, auditory discrimination, auditory pattern recognition, temporal aspects of audition, auditory performance in competing acoustic signals, and auditory performance with degraded acoustic signals. (American Speech-Language-Hearing Association 2005, pp.1–2)

An invisible disability which randomly prevents the sufferer from processing auditory (verbal) information. (Medical Research Council Institute of Hearing Research 2004)

Auditory processing is what we do with what we hear. (Katz, Stecker and Henderson 1992, pp.3–8)

Theory and research

A considerable body of research exists on specific learning difficulties, especially dyslexia, in normally hearing children, encompassing the biological, neurological, psychological and educational aspects of the disorder, along with approaches to remediation. However, even in hearing children there is very little high-quality outcome research to guide choices of intervention. A wide variety of interventions has been tried, and a handful of randomized controlled trials can be found in the literature. For example, Hatcher *et al.* (2006) report the results of a small group reading intervention for children who are delayed in their development of reading (not specifically diagnosed as dyslexic) at the end of their first year in school. They found improvements in measures of letter knowledge, single word reading and phoneme awareness in around three-quarters of children in the intervention group compared with the waiting-list controls. Using a sample of 98 primary-school-aged poor readers with persistent primary reflexes (those reflexes normally present during foetal and neonatal life), McPhillips, Hepper and Mulhern (2000) employed a randomized, double-blind placebo-controlled design to investigate the impact of practising specific movement sequences. Children in the experimental group achieved clinically significant gains in reading scores, which were greater than in the 'no movements' and 'non-specific movements' groups. Other interventions have included fatty acid treatment (e.g. Richardson 2004) and using coloured filters when reading (e.g. O'Connor *et al.* 1990), in children identified as having dyslexia or significant reading disabilities, with positive results. To our knowledge there are currently no published randomized controlled trials of interventions for dyspraxia or auditory processing disorders.

In hearing-impaired children the situation is considerably worse in terms of the available evidence – there is very little basic research on SLDs and no well-designed, large-scale intervention studies. At the present time, research in this area is at the stage of developing and evaluating teaching strategies for literacy, numeracy and science in hearing-impaired children generally, rather than those who are experiencing greater than anticipated difficulties learning, or who may be considered to have dyslexia. For example, in a recent survey of the literature, websites of professional organizations and education websites of American states, Easterbrooks and Stephensen (2006) identified a number of 'best practices' in educating deaf and hard of hearing students. The majority of these best practices were found to be based on 'developing research bases' rather than systematic outcome research.

Dyslexia

Knowledge and understanding about the causes of dyslexia have increased considerably in recent years. It is now accepted that dyslexia is an inherited condition, with a link between the disorder and regions on chromosome 6 (e.g. Francks *et al.* 2004; Grigorenko *et al.* 2003) and even evidence for the involvement of specific genes (Cope *et al.* 2005). There are identifiable differences in the brain structure and 'wiring' of people with dyslexia, and functional MRI studies have shown that people with dyslexia use a different part of their brain when reading compared with non-dyslexic people. Although the main focus is typically on literacy skills, individuals who are dyslexic may present with a range of difficulties in addition to the classic reading and spelling difficulties. For example, they often show poor handwriting skills, confusion over directionality (left-right, up-down), difficulty with sequencing steps in a task, and poor rote memory of numbers, names, unrelated facts or dates. The neurological differences/deficits in the brains of dyslexic people fundamentally lead to a lack of phonemic awareness (phonemes are the smallest unit of *spoken* language) resulting in problems distinguishing and manipulating sounds in spoken words. This is evidenced in poor performance on tasks such as phoneme segmentation, deletion, matching and substitution, and sound blending and rhyming tasks. Following on from this are difficulties with phonics and phonological processing – the correspondence between speech and written sounds, how written letters blend together to produce words, how letter sounds change according to the letters surrounding them, and other linguistic rules.

Clearly, any child who does not have adequate access to speech sounds through audition is likely to experience some degree of difficulty with phonemic awareness and phonic processing. For example, Sterne and Goswami (2000) report that deaf children can develop phonological awareness but that their phonological skills lag behind those of hearing children, and may develop in different ways. Briscoe, Bishop and Norbury (2001) found that children with mild–moderate sensori-neural hearing loss achieved significantly poorer scores on tests of phonological short-term memory, phonological discrimination and phonological awareness than age-matched hearing peers. However, these findings were *not* associated with clinically significant deficits in wider language and literacy abilities in the hearing-impaired children. Transler, Gombert and Leybaert (2001) presented data from severely and profoundly deaf children showing that those children with good speech abilities had greater awareness of phonics than those with poor speech abilities. Recently, Gibbs (2004) also provided evidence that children with moderate sensori-neural hearing loss can achieve similar reading levels to their hearing peers, but their phonological awareness skills are less well developed. What does appear to be a consistent finding is that there is a relationship between literacy attainment and degree of hearing loss, such that the more severe the hearing loss, the poorer the literacy achievement (see Mayberry 2002).

The 'Achievements of Deaf Pupils in Scotland' (ADPS 2006) project reported an incidence of dyslexia amongst deaf school-aged children attending units for hearing-impaired children between 2000 and 2004 of 90 in 5197 (1.7%), across the range of severity of difficulties. This is not dissimilar to the prevalence figures for the general population of around 4 per cent being classified as severely dyslexic (Badian 1984), but significantly less than suggested by Pennington (1991) of up to 10 per cent of children being dyslexic to some degree. The main problems in obtaining accurate figures are the differing definitions of dyslexia, varying cut-off points for severity and a multitude of possible assessments protocols. It is also probable that only the most severely affected children were identified in the ADPS project, due to difficulties gaining a formal diagnosis in this group.

Dyspraxia

Praxis, the ability to organize actions in new and creative ways rather than automatically, requires three interdependent stages – ideation, motor planning and execution. All these depend on the nerves around the body and within the brain sending the correct messages along the right pathways, at the right time and in the right order. Praxis develops from infancy throughout childhood as the child explores his or her environment, testing the consequences of actions, gradually repeating and refining them, until they become easy, smooth and automatic. Eventually many actions, including those involved in speech and language, require little or no praxis. In the child with developmental dyspraxia, this state is not achieved in the normal manner – there is a neurological deficit or malfunction that interferes with this process. However, despite extensive research over many years, little remains known about the exact aetiology of developmental dyspraxia. Some possible causes include insult to the developing foetus through infection, lack of oxygen momentarily at birth, failure of nerve cells or chemicals such as neurotransmitters to develop properly before birth and afterwards. There appears to be a tendency for similar neurological disorders to run in families. As yet, no strong evidence exists to support one hypothesis over another.

In the general, normally hearing population, the prevalence of developmental dyspraxia has been reported as 6 per cent of children aged 5–11 years to varying degrees (American Psychiatric Association 1994), but other estimates are as high as 20 per cent. The Dyspraxia Foundation provides figures of 10 per cent for all degrees of the disorder, and 2 per cent with a severe disorder. What is clear is that often only for those children in whom the difficulties are very marked is a diagnosis typically made. This is important in terms of identifying dyspraxia in deaf children, as, in common with other specific learning difficulties, difficulties may be attributed to the child's deafness, rather than the possibility of an additional disorder being considered. Only when difficulties are very obviously dyspraxic in nature are they assessed and intervention offered. To date, the only reported research on the incidence of dyspraxia in hearing-impaired children comes from the APDS project cited earlier, which found that 1.7 per cent of school-aged deaf children were dyspraxic. Equally, there is very little research on the relationship between dyspraxia and deafness, or on diagnosing dyspraxia in deaf children. The exception is research by van Uden (1983), Aplin (1987) and Broesterhuizen (1997) who examined the relationship between a variety of motor, memory and speech skills, suggesting that certain eupraxic skills (the normally developed automatic or coordinated movements) are predictive of some speech and reading skills in deaf children. Their findings do not form a cohesive pattern and therefore, as yet, there is no empirically based simple set of diagnostic tests for dyspraxia in hearing-impaired children.

Auditory processing disorder (APD)

Until 2000, the term central auditory processing disorder (CAPD) was commonly used, rather then APD. However, at the Bruton Conference in America, it was agreed that the emphasis should not be solely on the higher level, 'central' processes during which sound is interpreted; APD may be associated with difficulties in higher-order language, learning, memory or communication functions, but APD is not the *result* of these deficits (American Speech-Language-Hearing Association 2005). Research from cognitive neuroscience, neuropsychology and related areas indicates that a definition involving deficits in the auditory modality alone is neurophysiologically untenable, given the evidence that the central nervous system (CNS) encodes and manipulates sensory information in an interdependent, integrated fashion. However, for a diagnosis of APD, it is reasonable to expect a pattern of difficulties that is most pronounced in the auditory modality, or possibly auditory-specific in some individuals.

Whilst individuals with APD have difficulty processing sound at the most basic level (i.e. non-speech sounds), clearly, as sounds become more complex, deficits in processing are likely to become more apparent. Thus, APD is frequently associated with a range of other disorders, including reading and spelling difficulties (it is considered by some the underlying aetiology of dyslexia), speech and language disorders, ADHD and learning difficulties. It has also been discussed in relation to Asperger's syndrome, autism, Alzheimer's disease and traumatic brain injury. The aetiology of APD is not fully understood, but may be linked to delays in the maturation of the CNS, variations in the organization of the CNS or disease processes, and for some there may be a strong genetic element. Importantly for our area of interest (i.e. hearing-impaired children), auditory deprivation is considered by some to be a potential cause of APD.

Central auditory function can be assessed objectively using an electrophysiological index of the ability to discriminate speech sounds – the mismatch negativity (MMN) paradigm. The MMN is an automatic brain response to changes in the frequency, duration or intensity of a sound, or when one phoneme is replaced by another. This response has been found to differ significantly in children diagnosed with APD compared with normally developing children. Although its utility in children with a profound, bilateral hearing loss may be limited, the MMN paradigm has been found to be useful in assessing the central auditory function of children with cochlear implants. Although not widely available as a clinical tool, the procedure is likely to be a useful test as part of an assessment battery for APD, for example in deaf children with implants who are not making the anticipated progress in developing listening, language or literacy skills.

Sharma *et al.* (2006) compared the auditory processing of children with a reading disorder with a control group of children and found significant differences in MMN responses. They also reported significant correlations between reading fluency and most of the measures of APD they employed, leading them to conclude that children with reading disorders are also likely to have auditory processing disorders. It is also interesting to note that the MMN response has been found to distinguish very premature babies (tested at four years of age) from full-term children, and the degree of deviance of MMN response was associated with object-naming ability (Jansson-Verkasalo *et al.* 2003). Given that prematurity is a relatively common cause of deafness, we might expect this particular group of children to be at especially high risk of APD and language-learning difficulties.

There is little information regarding the epidemiology of APD. The prevalence of APD in children has been estimated to be 2–3 per cent (Chermak and Musiek 1997), and it appears to be more common in boys. However, this may be an underestimate, given that it is thought to co-exist frequently with other disorders such as speech and language disorder or delay, dyslexia, attention deficit disorder and social and/or emotional problems.

It is now generally accepted that children can have both a peripheral hearing loss and an APD (Chermak 2001), and indeed the presence of a hearing loss may place a child at risk for APD (a history of persistent otitis media is common in children diagnosed with APD). The auditory pathways and centres in the brain develop as they are stimulated with sound, so if the range of sounds is limited in some way, optimal development of the system may not be able to occur, resulting in auditory processing deficits.

Assessment of specific learning difficulties

For most SLDs, multi-disciplinary assessment is highly desirable, if not essential. It is useful to have the input of a paediatrician or a doctor with an interest in audiology (e.g. an audiological physician), who can provide information on the child's medical history and any relevant diagnoses. For example, significant prematurity is often associated with problems with attention skills. This sort of information is important, not only from the point of view of diagnosing an SLD, but also in terms of the practicalities of assessing the child.

Assessment of the child's speech and language by a speech and language therapist specializing in childhood deafness is very important for most types of SLD, and may in fact be the trigger for assessment by a psychologist. In particular, the diagnosis of dyspraxia, especially oro-motor dyspraxia, may be made primarily by a speech and language therapist, with psychology taking a very supplementary role. Other members of the multi-disciplinary team may include a teacher of the deaf and an audiological scientist, depending on the nature of the presenting difficulties. The teacher of the deaf can provide useful information regarding the child's academic progress and their behaviour and learning style in the school setting. The expertise of an audiological scientist and/or audiological physician is essential where a diagnosis of central auditory processing disorder is being considered, as most of the tests required are audiological.

General considerations

The first consideration when planning the assessment of SLDs in a hearing-impaired child is that it can be a very time-consuming process. It is essential to find out as much as you can about the child's language skills before meeting them for the assessment so that you can make some (tentative) guesses as to which tests may be useful and appropriate, and those that may be beyond the child's current language levels, making administration unreliable. It is also advisable to discuss the child's difficulties with their school teachers and speech and language therapist (if they have one), as they typically have a very good idea of the nature of the difficulties.

Most standardized tests used by psychologists involve verbal instructions, and may require verbal responses from the child. In many cases, the child does not have the language skills necessary to understand the instructions fully if presented in the standardized manner stated in the test's manual. However, if the test can be administered with some modification (for example using sign to supplement speech, or writing instructions down), but without substantively altering the task or deviating too far from the standardized administration, the results can yield some useful information. However, in this sort of scenario, results cannot be interpreted using the test's norms, and should be done with caution. Pragmatically, it is probably better to simplify instructions, for example in terms of sentence structure or length, or the vocabulary used, rather than stick rigidly to the manual's instructions and then have to abandon a test the child could tackle because they have misunderstood what they need to do. It is always important to allow the child sufficient time to process verbal information, and to check comprehension at regular intervals.

In terms of the test room itself, there are a few important points to bear in mind. Good lighting is essential, as many hearing-impaired children gain a lot of clues about speech from lip-reading, and this is more difficult in low light or if the speaker's face is in shadow. Also, the speaker's face should be clearly visible to the child, and for this reason it is usually better to sit opposite the child rather than next to them or diagonally across the table from them. As with any child being tested, the assessor will need to judge whether the child is likely to cooperate or perform better with or without the parent(s)/carer(s) present in the room, and negotiate this sensitively with all concerned.

Steps/procedure for information gathering

Before administering any tests, a full history and background information should be obtained from the child's parents or primary caregiver. A summary of the main areas to be covered is given below, but any other relevant information should also be noted:

- aetiology of hearing-impairment – congenital, syndromic, progressive, meningitis

- degree of hearing loss and language development

- brief medical history – prematurity, major illness, medication

- early development – milestones, feeding, play

- family history – especially reading, spelling, speech/language difficulties

- cultural background including languages used in the home

- siblings – any similar difficulties

- schooling – communication mode, peer relationships, academic achievement/attainment levels, social development

- behaviour – attention problems, oppositional behaviour and so on, across contexts.

Assessment of non-verbal cognitive abilities

The first step in an assessment of SLDs, arguably for every child, is an assessment of his or her non-verbal cognitive abilities. This allows global learning difficulties to be excluded as a cause for the child's lack of progress. It may also identify specific areas of weakness within the child's non-verbal profile, for example specific difficulties with visual patterns (e.g. ♣♦♥♣♦♥? ?) and sequences (e.g. ○ ○ ○ ?).

In a hearing child the Performance sub-tests of the WISC IVUK (Wechsler 2004), or the British Ability Scales II (Elliot, Smith and McCulloch 1996) are typically used to assess non-verbal abilities. However, as mentioned earlier, these tests rely heavily on the child's ability to understand verbal instructions that may be quite complex, and if the test is administered strictly according to the directions, it allows no variation in the words used and little or no repetition. Therefore, use of a test specifically designed to be employed with children with limited language skills is preferable, unless the child has well-established oral language skills. This also has the advantage of making the child feel comfortable in the test situation and achieve to his or her potential. Two such tests are commonly available, the Leiter International Performance Scale – Revised (Leiter-R; Roid and Miller 1997), and the Snijders-Oomen Non-Verbal Intelligence Test (SON-R; Snijders, Tellegen and Laros 1989; Tellegen et al. 1998). Both comprise a number of sub-tests assessing a variety of visual reasoning abilities. The Leiter-R is particularly useful in that it also includes a series of visual memory and attention sub-tests, including a visual memory span task.

If the results of the non-verbal assessment indicate that the child's IQ is below 70, in other words is in the range defined as indicating generalized learning difficulties, it is inadvisable to test further, or attempt to diagnose an SLD. It would be almost impossible to determine whether the child had specific difficulties on top of the global ones, and in terms of formal diagnosis based on ICD-10 guidelines, the global difficulties 'trump' specific difficulties. In this situation it would be extremely difficult to convince the relevant authorities that remedial intervention should focus on any one area.

Assessment of specific types of learning difficulties

Usually, the referring agent will have given some indication of the type of learning difficulty they think the child may be experiencing, even if only in broad terms such as reading, sequencing, mathematical or memory difficulties. This, along with the results of the general non-verbal assessment, will guide the choice of further tests to use. However, it is important not to rely too heavily on this approach as it may close the mind to other possibilities. In the following sections are some suggestions of tests that may be useful for diagnosing some SLDs in hearing-impaired children. However, there are many tests, or sub-scales of tests that perform the same function, and therefore may be substituted, and not all will be listed here.

Developmental dyslexia

Here the aim is to establish whether the child's reading and spelling attainments are significantly delayed/poorer in relation to their non-verbal ability, *over-and-above* the deficit to be expected given the degree of hearing-impairment. In addition, for a diagnosis of dyslexia to be made with confidence there should be evidence of a further discrepancy between the child's achieved reading level and their phonemic awareness and phonetic decoding abilities. Clearly this is a very challenging judgement to attempt to make, given that the child's access to speech sounds will have been distorted to a greater or lesser extent, and their own speech production may not be clear. Therefore, testing should only be done by a person experienced in working with hearing-impaired children, and help may need to be enlisted from the parents to 'interpret' the child's responses, if necessary. The following behavioural manifestations of dyslexia may be noted as part of the history including:

- difficulties remembering rhymes as a pre-schooler

- relatively short attention span

- sequencing problems (e.g. coloured beads)

- jumbling letters of whole words in speech, for example par cark

- problems with physical skills such as catching, throwing and kicking a ball, skipping, hopping

- marked, unexpected difficulty with reading and spelling

- mixing up of directional words, for example up/down, in/out, left/right

- writing letters and/or numbers the wrong way around

- leaving letters out of written words

- difficulty with rote learning, for example times tables, the alphabet, days of the week in order.

TESTS FOR DYSLEXIA

Below is a list of possible tests that may be helpful; it is neither exhaustive, nor should every test be administered as many serve the same function.

Literacy attainments: reading

- Wechlser Objective Reading Dimensions (WORD; Wechsler 1993). This is a well-established test widely used among hearing children, giving three sub-scales (Basic Reading, Spelling and Comprehension) and a composite score. The Comprehension sub-scale is probably the least useful for hearing-impaired children. It has recently been superseded by the Wechsler Individual Achievement Test (WIAT II; Wechsler 2005), which includes three tests of reading – Word Reading, Reading Comprehension and Pseudoword Decoding.

- Neale Analysis of Reading Ability, Second Edition (Neale 1997). In this test the Supplementary Diagnostic Tests are particularly useful in beginner readers.

- Test of Word Reading Efficiency (TOWRE; Torgesen, Wagner and Rashotte 1999). The first sub-test in this test assesses the child's ability to read 'sight' words as fast they can.

Language abilities

- Weschler Intelligence Scale for Children IV[UK] (WISC IV[UK]; Wechsler 2004). The Similarities and Vocabulary sub-tests are useful here to get an idea of language abilities where reading or writing skills are not needed.

Phonetic decoding abilities

- Graded Non-word Reading Test (Snowling, Slothard and McLean 1996).

- TOWRE. The second sub-test assesses the ability to use decoding skills to read real words.

Phonological processing (phonemic awareness)

- Phonological Assessment Battery (PhAB; Frederickson, Frith and Reason 1999). This battery comprises tests of naming speed, non-word reading and a rhyme test.

- Comprehensive Test of Phonological Processing (CTOPP; Wagner, Torgesen and Rashotte 1999). Assesses phoneme segmentation, speed of phonological processing (rapid letter, number, picture naming) and phoneme blending.

Other

- Short-term verbal memory span – digit span sub-test from the WISC IV^{UK}.

Case example: Dyslexia

Thomas is 11:6 years old. He received a cochlear implant at the age of three years. Regular audiological testing and assessments showed that he was making good progress in terms of listening skills and discrimination of speech sounds. His hearing levels with the cochlear implant were around 35–40dBHL (decibel hearing level) across the speech frequencies; the profound loss remained unchanged in his non-implanted ear. Concerns were raised by Thomas's teacher of the deaf, and the speech and language therapist from the cochlear implant programme who assessed his progress, that his literacy skills were not as expected given his hearing levels and listening skills. The following test results were accumulated over three sessions:

Leiter-R

Full Non-verbal IQ	106 (mean = 100)	
Fluid Reasoning Composite	112 (mean = 100)	
Spatial Visualization Composite	107 (mean = 100)	
Forward Visual Memory Span	13 (mean = 10)	
Reverse Visual Memory Span	14 (mean = 10)	
Sustained Visual Attention	13 (mean = 10)	

WORD

Basic Reading	70 (mean = 100)	Age Equivalent 7:0
Spelling	67 (mean = 100)	Age Equivalent 7:0

WISC III^{UK}	
Similarities	Age Equivalent 9:9
Vocabulary	Age Equivalent 6:0
Graded Non-word Reading Test	Age Equivalent 5:6
CTOPP	
Phoneme Segmentation	Age Equivalent 5:0
Speed of Phonological Processing	Age Equivalent 7:8
Phoneme Blending	Age Equivalent 6:8
Short-term Verbal Memory Span	Age Equivalent 8:2

These results indicate that Thomas is making very slow progress in learning to read and spell, and that his phoneme awareness and phonetic decoding abilities are significantly below his reading level. This, taking into account his history of access to speech sounds, is highly indicative of developmental dyslexia.

Developmental dyspraxia

There are two primary presentations of dyspraxia – a generalized motor dyspraxia involving both gross and fine motor skills, and verbal, or articulatory dyspraxia where the main difficulties are in the areas of speech and expressive language. Children may show signs of either or both forms of the disorder.

One of the most important steps in diagnosing dyspraxia in hearing-impaired children is to eliminate other possible causes of motor difficulties, for example those related to specific aetiologies of deafness, or medical and neurological disorders. Therefore, a paediatrician's and/or neurologist's evaluation of the child is essential. Assessment by specialist speech and language therapists, occupational therapists and clinical or educational psychologists is also important, to build up a comprehensive picture of the child's skills and difficulties. One of the aims of assessment is to distinguish dyspraxia from other language disorders or delay, and therefore, where possible, it is useful to have a general assessment of language skills. If this is not possible, perhaps because the child's oral/aural language skills are too limited to allow standardized tests to be administered, diagnosis of dyspraxia may be made on the basis of comprehensive assessment of other areas, but with cautious interpretation. As usual, it is important to place any difficulties within the context of the child's developmental level and overall cognitive functioning, and be aware of the possibility that these difficulties may have had a negative impact on self-esteem and social relationships. Information from the child's teacher(s), in addition to that from his or her parents is very important, as many of the 'symptoms' of dyspraxia are primarily apparent in the school context. A variety of psychometric tests can be used to provide information about a child's strengths and areas of difficulty and to provide supporting 'evidence' for the diagnosis. However, in the case of verbal dyspraxia, the primary method of diagnosing the disorder is through careful analysis of a sample of the child's speech, preferably videotaped, by a speech and language therapist who is familiar with the normal articulation patterns of hearing-impaired children. A child with dyspraxia may exhibit a range of behavioural manifestations of the disorder including difficulty:

- hopping, jumping, catching a ball
- dressing, using buttons and zips
- holding a pencil properly
- doing jigsaws
- pouring without spilling
- copying from the blackboard
- using scissors
- writing neatly and drawing
- making speech sounds, sequencing them in words and sentences (intelligibility)
- controlling breathing when speaking
- controlling pitch, intonation and rhythm in speech
- learning to blow their nose
- feeding as a baby
- reading and spelling
- anxiety and distractibility, frustration and poor peer relationships.

TESTS FOR DYSPRAXIA
General motor skills

- Bruininks-Oseretsky Test of Motor Proficiency, Second Edition (Bruininks and Bruininks 2005). Provides composite scores covering fine motor control, manual coordination, body coordination, strength and agility and a total motor composite, for children and young adults aged 4–21 years.

- Movement Assessment Battery for Children (Movement ABC; Henderson and Sugden 1992). This test provides screening, assessment and remediation/management programmes for children with movement problems aged 4–12 years.

- Wide Range Assessment of Visual-Motor Abilities (WRAVMA; Adams and Sheslow 1995). This test assesses visuo-motor integration, visual-spatial and fine motor skills in children and young adults aged 3–17 years.

With each of these tests, it may be necessary to translate instructions into BSL, or demonstrate or model to the hearing-impaired child what they are required to do, if they have difficulty understanding the spoken instructions.

Speech and language abilities

- Clinical Evaluation of Language Fundamentals, Fourth Edition UK (Semel, Wiig and Secord 2006). Four core sub-tests can be used to derive a Total Language Score, to obtain a general impression of the child's language skills.

- Reynell Developmental Language Scales III (Edwards et al. 1997). This test comprises two scales (Comprehension and Expression), with a number of sub-tests in each. It is a comprehensive, lengthy test, and some sub-tests are more useful and appropriate than others for hearing-impaired children.

- Wechsler Intelligence Scale for Children IV (WISC IV^{UK}; Wechsler 2004). Where a comprehensive assessment of language has not been possible, the Similarities and Vocabulary sub-tests can give a guide to the child's level of language ability.

- Diagnostic Evaluation of Articulation and Phonology (DEAP; Dodd et al. 2002). This test is useful in assessing children (aged 3–6:11) suspected of having oro-motor dyspraxia. It evaluates articulation and phonological processes, along with oro-motor ability, and includes a diagnostic screen.

When using tests of language ability with hearing-impaired children it must be emphasized that interpreting and reporting the results should be done with great care: these tests have not been standardized on hearing-impaired children and therefore comparison with norms derived from hearing children may be misleading. Nevertheless, using these tests can be very informative, as they do provide an indication of what the child is able to do, including highlighting inconsistencies between different areas of language skills (e.g. comprehension versus expressive vocabulary). Test results can also be used to monitor progress, when changes within the same individual are more important than comparison with other individuals, hearing or deaf.

Executive function/organization skills

- Behaviour Rating Inventory of Executive Function (BRIEF; Gioia *et al.* 2000). This questionnaire has two versions – parent and teacher – and can provide useful information about the child's working memory, self-control, flexibility and ability to plan and organize, with norms for children and young adults aged 5–18 years.

Auditory processing disorder

An auditory processing problem may be suspected in a hearing-impaired child whose loss is within the mild to moderate range, or in a child with a cochlear implant, who appears to be making poorer progress in developing language and literacy skills than expected given their access to sounds, including speech sounds. They may be experiencing difficulties in the classroom, despite good acoustic conditions, small class sizes and appropriate support from staff trained specifically to work with deaf children.

It is essential that a multi-disciplinary team undertake the assessment for APD, with the major role adopted by audiologists. Speech and language therapists also need to be involved, with psychologists potentially contributing relatively little in terms of formal psychometric assessment. A global learning difficulty or cognitive deficit needs to be excluded, as does a higher-order speech or language problem. Other diagnoses such as attention deficit hyperactivity disorder or Asperger's syndrome may also need to be considered, and investigated. Auditory neuropathy and auditory dys-synchrony also need to be ruled out by audiologists as possible causes of the child's listening difficulties. Psychologists will also need to focus on assessing the social, emotional and behavioural needs of the child, to build a comprehensive picture of the impact of the child's difficulties, particularly to inform intervention plans. Audiological testing should focus on non-speech sounds to control for cognitive and linguistic demands, and memory load, so that any deficit identified is truly due to auditory processing problems. It is also important that the motor response required for the tests does not confound results.

At present, it is very difficult to diagnose APD in a child less than seven years of age due to the tests available, both in terms of the established norms, and the task requirements. Currently, electrophysiological tests such as MMN and P300 are the only options in younger children, and these have very limited availability in the UK. However, ongoing research conducted by the Medical Research Council Institute of Hearing Research (MRC IHR) is developing and validating a battery of tests suitable for children as young as three years of age, incorporating a computerized, visually appealing test of frequency discrimination, which will hopefully be useful in all but the most profoundly deaf children.

Ideally, assessment for APD should include comparison of auditory processing tasks with analogous tasks in another sensory modality, for example visual processing, so that it can be established whether any processing deficits are auditory or more generalized. However, it is not a necessary condition for the deficits to be modality-specific for a diagnosis of APD to be made. Visual memory and attention tasks are useful for this purpose. APD may be manifested behaviourally in the following ways including difficulties:

- hearing in noisy situations

- following long conversations

- remembering spoken information or instructions, particularly where there are multiple components/steps

- maintaining attention if other sounds are present – easily distracted by irrelevant sounds

- with organizational skills

- directing, sustaining or dividing attention

- reading and/or spelling.

TESTS FOR APD
Audiological assessment

- Behavioural/psychoacoustic tests: Pure tone audiometry; speech in noise; temporal processing, for example pitch or duration pattern perception; binaural integration, for example dichotic listening for digits (not generally possible in children with cochlear implants); sound localization; backward and simultaneous masking; temporal integration.

- Electroacoustic tests: Immittance measures, otoacoustic emissions.

- Electrophysiologic tests: Auditory brainstem-evoked responses; P300; MMN.

Cognitive assessment

- General cognitive ability: Leiter-R (Roid and Miller 1997) or SON-R (Snijders *et al.* 1989; Tellegen *et al.* 1998)

- Memory: Digit span, forward and reverse; visual memory span, for example from the Leiter-R, forward and reverse.

Language assessment

- Receptive and expressive language: Reynell Developmental Language Scales III (Edwards *et al.* 1997).

- Reading ability: WORD (Wechsler 1993) or Neale Analysis of Reading Ability (Neale 1997).

- Repetition of nonsense words: NEPSY (Korkman, Kirk and Kemp 1998).

- Phonological processing: CTOPP (Wagner *et al.* 1999), PhAB (Frederickson *et al.* 1999).

Where there is a sensori-neural hearing loss the choice of audiological tests should focus on those most resistant to the effects of a peripheral loss, using stimuli that are minimally affected. For example, tonal or other non-verbal stimuli, or verbal stimuli with high linguistic redundancy may be used. It may also be possible to administer the P300 test. In addition, if the hearing loss is less severe at certain frequencies, behavioural and electrophysiological tests should be administered using stimuli at those frequencies. Further details of testing hearing-impaired children for APD are given in the American Speech-Language-Hearing Association (2005) technical report on APDs.

Conclusions

Understanding of specific learning difficulties in hearing-impaired children is in its infancy. There is little empirical evidence in the field and no established, agreed methods for assessing or diagnosing SLDs in this group. Despite this, we would argue that many hearing-impaired children do experience difficulties in addition to their deafness that can be construed in a manner comparable to SLDs in hearing children. The suggestions we have made regarding possible tests for dyslexia, dyspraxia and APD are based on clinical experience of what works in practice, and are therefore likely to evolve over time. We would always advocate attempting to use well-established, reliable and valid psychometric assessments, although interpreting the results in hearing-impaired children for whom there are no norms, must be approached with some caution. Building a coherent, consistent picture of the child's difficulties may take considerable time, or may never be fully achieved. However, it is essential that the needs of these children are not overlooked, and that where there are concerns regarding a child's progress these are investigated in a timely fashion, and that specialist support and intervention are provided when necessary.

5 Disorders of Communication

'Communication disorders' is a broad term encompassing a range of difficulties, and may be used to include disorders such as autistic spectrum disorders (ASD, autism, atypical autism and Asperger's syndrome), social communication disorder, pervasive developmental disorder (PDD) and specific language impairment or speech and language disorder. This variety provides a challenge when trying to define the difficulties of a particular child, as the choice of one diagnosis over others will have significant implications – for prognosis, intervention and education. Confusingly, the terms are used by some writers interchangeably, but by others as distinct categories. However, the most commonly used term is probably ASDs, which as the name suggests, implies that difficulties in this area occur along a spectrum, with some children only mildly affected and others with severe disabilities across all areas of functioning. The situation is further complicated by the fact that 'symptoms' indicative of a communication disorder may be present in a deaf child giving the impression that the child has a disorder, whereas in fact the communication behaviours are the result of late diagnosis of deafness, the communicative environment or possibly the communication mode, or other factors.

The main focus of this chapter will be on difficulties usually referred to as ASDs, although we will also briefly discuss specific disorders of language and social communication disorder, in terms of their presentation and assessment, in order to clarify the distinction between the three, and highlight the areas of overlap. Theoretical perspectives on ASDs will be presented, with consideration of their relevance to hearing-impaired children, both with and without ASDs.

Research in this area will be summarized, including the literature on intervention outcome studies. The remainder of the chapter will consider approaches to the assessment of ASDs in deaf children in some depth, as this is fundamental to providing appropriate support and intervention to families of a deaf child with autism. This will be supported by the presentation of an extended case example to illustrate the process.

Deafness or communication disorder?

When a deaf child is referred to mental health or psychology services because of concerns about his or her development or use of communication and language, it can be very difficult to distinguish between variations due to exposure to language and communication, and those due to an underlying problem in these areas. This is especially the case at the 'mild' end of the spectrum where difficulties may be subtle and a wide variety of factors may be influencing the child's learning of language – age at diagnosis of deafness, degree of hearing loss, mode of communication, parental communicative efficacy, parental mental health and so on. In the next two sections, speech and language, and social communication disorder will be described along with some brief suggestions for assessment procedures, which can then be contrasted with the presentation and assessment of autistic spectrum disorder later in the chapter.

Specific disorders of speech and language; language disorders

Language disorders can present themselves within the domains of expressive, receptive or mixed disorders. A language disorder includes difficulties with speech processing and production (phonology), understanding word meaning (semantics), and poor grammatical knowledge or sentence use (syntactic or morphological). Difficulties are also seen in the integration of language and context (decoding meaning) and understanding intended meaning (social communication and pragmatics). Also, in some children, there can be a disorder of the speech system (production).

Disorders of articulation in the absence of any other difficulties are evidenced by omissions of words in speech, distortions, substitutions and inconsistencies in pronunciation. Expressive language disorder is characterized by a restricted vocabulary, word substitutions, omissions of word endings and prefixes, syntactical errors and short sentences. Hearing children with a receptive language disorder will show lack of understanding of grammatical structure (for example negatives, questions and comparatives), difficulty following instructions, and also significant delay in expressive language. Non-verbal communication, including gesture, mime, demonstration and non-speech vocalizations are usually normal (World Health Organization 1992). However, therein lies the problem. The speech and verbal comprehension of hearing-impaired children is often characterized by errors of the kind described above, when there is no additional language disorder. The non-verbal communication of deaf children may not be completely typical of their hearing peers, but again this does not necessarily mean that they have a language, or any other, disorder. Also, language disorders are frequently associated with social, emotional and behavioural problems in hearing children, but there is a high rate of these difficulties in deaf children, even without language disorders. Thus, distinguishing between the normal variations of the language (and behaviour) of hearing-impaired children, and the language (and behaviour) of a hearing-impaired child with a language disorder is very complex. Deaf children may find it difficult to behave appropriately in unpredictable situations, for example social situations with peers, as they are not able to read the social cues easily and thus decode meaning that is not explicitly shared. As young children, they may hit out (possibly as an attempt to interact) or withdraw (maybe preferring to play on their own) (Fujiki *et al.* 1999). Thus, understanding the rules of social communication will be difficult, as seen in the learning of turn-taking in toddlers.

ASSESSMENT OF LANGUAGE DISORDERS

Assessment in a hearing-impaired child is in many respects the same as in a hearing child, although the professionals involved should be experienced in communicating with and assessing hearing-impaired children. The rationale underlying assessment can be summarized as follows:

- In accordance with diagnostic guidelines, language disorders must be assessed in the context of expectations appropriate for the child's 'mental age', or more specifically their non-verbal cognitive abilities (see Chapter 4 for more information on this).

- A detailed developmental history should always be taken, and videotaping the informal interactions and formal language assessment is helpful for subsequent detailed analysis of the child's language.

- In the absence of specific criteria, the clinician then has to decide, largely on the basis of experience, whether the child's language is sufficiently more delayed or disordered than would be anticipated given their degree of hearing loss and their non-verbal cognitive abilities, to warrant a diagnosis of language disorder.

Diagnosis is particularly difficult in hearing-impaired children, as language delays resulting from the deafness may 'mask' difficulties, which in a hearing child would be categorized as specific language disorders. The range of psychometric tests that can be used in hearing-impaired children is limited and interpreting the results is complex. A few standardized assessment batteries do present some normative data, usually on a small sample, for hearing-impaired children, but this assumes that it has been possible to administer the tests in the first place, as many deaf children do not have the verbal language or literacy skills needed to understand and follow the instructions, or respond verbally. Although it is sometimes possible to use sign language for both the administration and response mode, this typically makes the test very difficult to score, and more particularly, difficult to interpret the results. Hence, assessment frequently falls into the qualitative domain, with supporting evidence from standardized tests. Standardized findings alone should not be used without clinical information, bearing in mind the context from which it has been derived, for example the clinic setting, home or educational environment, in familiar versus novel and formal versus informal settings.

One useful approach to gathering information about a deaf child's language and communication is a play-based assessment (Linder 1993). The child's general development, social interaction, communicative intent and behaviour can all be observed in this way. Play items should include a range of toys, aimed at both younger and older children than the child being assessed, using a range of skill domains, for example drawing, puzzles, doll play, tea set, small world people and animals, construction, shape-sorter, lotto game, dressing up items.

Given the need to demonstrate that the child's difficulties are in excess of what would be expected given their general developmental level or level of intellectual functioning, it is important to obtain a measure of these. The use of a test of non-verbal performance is therefore key in the assessment of a specific language disorder. One such scale, the Leiter International Performance Scale – Revised (Leiter-R; Roid and Miller 1997) provides a comprehensive assessment of the visual perception, reasoning, memory and attention skills of children and from two years upwards, which is suitable for use with children with a hearing-impairment. Roid and Miller (1997) provide standardized scores for deaf children, although these are based on a relatively small sample, and it is not altogether clear from the information provided whether the sample is representative of hearing-impaired children generally.

When assessing for a language disorder, as with any of the communication disorders, it is important that professionals work in a team. The input of a speech and language therapist specializing in deafness is necessary; they will be able to use standardized language tests, alongside observation of the child's skills across contexts. The significant difference between language disorder and social communication disorder or ASD is that when a child has a language disorder *the child will be sociable and want to communicate with others*. In contrast, children with an ASD typically show little desire to communicate and may actually become distressed if someone tries to interact with them when they are not 'ready', or in a manner that they find difficult to understand. Therefore, as mentioned above, it is important to see the child across settings, for example in their educational setting, home and clinic and over a period of time. The time factor enables the therapists to see a child's rate of development and progress, and gives the child time to get to know the assessors and therefore feel comfortable interacting with them. Therefore, when assessing a deaf child for the possibility of a speech and/or language disorder, the role of a psychologist may primarily be to assess non-verbal functioning and to rule out the possibility that the difficulties with language are part of a social communication disorder or ASD.

The following areas will need formal assessment by a speech and language therapist to make a diagnosis:

- speech processing (phonology) difficulties

- understanding of word meaning (vocabulary)

- grammatical knowledge and sentence structure

- difficulties with integrating language and context (decoding meaning)

- understanding of intended meaning (social communication/pragmatics).

Two major assumptions have been made throughout the above: that the child uses oral language rather than sign language, and that they have sufficient language abilities to tackle formal assessments, even if they are not administered in the standardized fashion intended. This said, it is possible for a child whose only language is manual to have a language disorder, but here you would need a fluent British Sign Language (BSL) user (and Deaf advocate where possible) to assist with the assessment, and use of an assessment of BSL abilities.

Social communication disorder

This descriptor is often used as a general name for children who present with difficulties with language, communication and social interaction. These children typically do not show the third area of the triad of difficulties in an autistic spectrum disorder – repetitive and specific interests – thus not meeting full criteria for the diagnosis of ASD. Social communication disorder is not classified in either of the current diagnostic and statistical manuals, *ICD-10* (World Health Organization 1992) or *DSM-IV* (American Psychiatric Association 1994). The diagnosis is thus descriptive only. However, difficulties of this sort could potentially be classified as 'atypical autism', which according to the *ICD-10* includes children whose impaired development only becomes manifest after three years of age, and/or there are abnormalities in only one or two of the three areas of functioning required for a diagnosis of autism (see later section for a full description of these).

A social communication disorder is characterized by:

- severe difficulties in the areas of language, communication and social interaction, but not meeting the full criteria for ASD

- language disorder plus additional difficulties with social and play skills (possibly with some adherence to routines but not meeting criteria for repetitive and specific interests)

- non-verbal learning and pre-verbal communication skills within the normal, non-learning disability range.

ASSESSMENT OF SOCIAL COMMUNICATION DISORDER

In deaf children, social communication difficulties are apparent when a child is struggling with the non-verbal aspects of communication as well as language. In this case, the child's verbal or signed language skills are of less importance than their pre-verbal and non-verbal communication skills, which will need to be assessed and include:

- eye contact

- pointing (using the index finger) with reflexive looking, that is, joint attention: looking at an object of interest then at the face of the other person, then back to the object, to share interest

- use of facial and bodily expressions to compensate for lack of language

- bringing items to share not just when help is needed

- smiling to another person to share pleasure

- responding to another person's smile at them.

Deaf children may have poorly developed skills in these areas for a variety of reasons that are unrelated to a social communication problem, as the following case example illustrates.

Case example: An impoverished social history

Rachel was referred for assessment by her health visitor, who was concerned about her development generally. At the age of two-and-a-half years she was not eating well and uninterested in feeding herself, and showed no signs of awareness of her toileting needs. On observation in the clinic, Rachel actively avoided interacting with any adults other than her mother, refusing to make eye contact despite much encouragement and the offer of a number of interesting activities. She spent much of the session with her face hidden in her mother's lap. When interacting with her mother, Rachel passively waited for toys to be handed to her, then appeared not to know what to do with them, quickly dropping them to the floor.

Rachel's mother described her circumstances as very stressful. She is a single-parent, with two other children, a son aged 14 years who had been excluded from school for violent behaviour and a five-year-old daughter with significant learning difficulties. Each child had a different father, none of whom contributed to the family either financially or emotionally. Rachel's mother said that she had little time to play with Rachel because of the needs of her other children, and had been unable to attend sign language classes for the same reason. She therefore felt helpless in communicating with Rachel, and had given up trying. She described feeling constantly exhausted and overwhelmed. She also said that she had been prescribed anti-depressants by her doctor, but felt that these were not helping much.

In Rachel's case it is possible that she has some form of ASD, and further assessment is certainly indicated. However, it is also possible that the communicative experiences, quality of attachment to her mother and the social circumstances to which she is subjected, are underlying her presentation of difficulties.

In terms of making a diagnosis, it is important to re-assess a child with a diagnosis of social communication disorder after a period of time, as it is possible that repetitive and specific interests become more apparent as a child develops and higher demands are placed on them, for example coping with the demands of the school environment, thus meeting the criteria for an autistic spectrum disorder. As with language disorders, the child should be assessed across settings and across time, and a non-verbal assessment will need to be carried out. In order to eliminate the possibility that a child meets the criteria for ASD, this diagnosis needs to be made by following the full assessment process for ASD.

Autistic spectrum disorder

Autism is considered a 'pervasive developmental disorder', which means that the disorder is present across every situation within which the child functions. It is manifest before the age of three years. Evidence of a triad of areas of dysfunction needs to be observed for the diagnosis to be made: abnormalities in reciprocal social interactions, communication and restricted, stereotyped or repetitive behaviours (World Health Organization 1992). General cognitive delay is usually also present. The observed behaviours in autistic spectrum disorder include poor understanding of socio-emotional cues, leading to a lack of, or inappropriate, responses to other people's emotions, poor use of social signals and lack of integration of social, emotional and communicative behaviours. There are also qualitative abnormalities in communication generally and impaired make-believe, social imitative and symbolic play. The other primary area of behaviour disturbance in autism lies in restricted, repetitive and stereo-typed patterns of behaviour, resulting in the child imposing rigidity and routine on a variety of play and other activities, any changes leading to anxiety and distress. Autistic children frequently have difficulties generalizing what they have learnt from one situation to another, and they may also experience difficulties in integrating information gained from the different sense modalities. In addition to these specific areas of difficulty, autistic children also frequently show a range of other problems, such as sleeping and eating difficulties, fears or phobias, temper tantrums and aggressive behaviour (World Health Organization 1992). Asperger's syndrome, considered by some as part of the autistic spectrum but by others as a separate entity, differs from autism in that there is no general delay in cognitive or language development. It is characterized by the same qualitative impairments in reciprocal social interactions and restricted, stereotyped, repetitive behaviours and interests as found in autism.

Autistic spectrum disorder – key points

- Triad of difficulties: social interaction, communication and restricted, repetitive, stereotyped behaviours.

- Triad is inconsistent with chronological age.

- Not all skills are below a two-year level.

- Asperger's diagnosis has implications for management (triad of difficulties is the same).

- Normal language development before three years of age, with no significant learning needs is required for Asperger's diagnosis.

Aetiology and epidemiology of ASD in the deaf population

The aetiology of autism, although much researched and debated, currently remains inadequately understood (Rutter 2005). There is strong evidence that genetic factors play an important role (e.g. Bailey *et al.* 1995), although no specific genes have yet been consistently identified. Therefore, it has been proposed that multiple genes interacting are responsible for the genetic complexity underlying the disorder (Risch *et al.* 1999).

Although genetic susceptibility or causation is likely, environmental risk factors may also play a role, including both in-utero and 'events' after birth, the most publicized 'cause' of autism of this nature being the measles, mumps and rubella vaccine. However, recent studies have ruled out such an association (e.g. Fombonne 2005). Thankfully, it is also no longer the case that mothers of autistic children are blamed for inducing the disorder in their children through being cold and unresponsive to their infants. For example, Buhrmann (1979, pp.724–727) began: 'Since this syndrome is always a manifestation of disturbed interpersonal relationships…'

An association between certain causes of deafness and autism has been noted by Jure, Rapin and Tuchman (1991), for example congenital rubella and cytomegalovirus infections, and syndromes such as CHARGE association. In these cases it can be hypothesized that the damage to the brain resulting from infection or generalized brain abnormalities gives rise to both the deafness and autistic symptoms. Interestingly, Jure *et al.* (1991) also noted that in the six deaf-autistic children with deaf siblings in their sample, none of the siblings were also autistic. This suggests that in these children the two disorders had separate aetiologies.

In their large-scale study of 1150 hearing-impaired children (Jure *et al.* 1991), the prevalence of ASD was 4 per cent. The gender difference was approximately 2:1 for boys:girls, the median age for detection of hearing loss was two years, and that for ASD diagnosis four years (22% were not diagnosed until very much later). Over 80 per cent of the children in the study had a severe to profound hearing loss, with 17 per cent having a known syndrome of which deafness was one symptom. Thirteen per cent of the sample had a hearing-impaired sibling; however, none of these siblings had autism. Additional disabilities were common: 35 per cent of the sample had visual difficulties, 17 per cent epilepsy and 24 per cent had 'hard' neurological signs. However, the authors acknowledge that their samples were drawn from biased populations, so it is important to stress that the deaf children in this study may not be representative of deaf children generally, or those typically presenting to ASD services. There appears to be a higher prevalence of additional difficulties, especially sensory, in this group, which is likely to be linked to the high rate of syndromic causes of the disabilities.

Currently, there is some debate over the true incidence of autism generally (i.e. not specifically in deaf children), questioning whether rates of autism are truly increasing or whether broadening of diagnostic concepts and criteria, increased awareness of the disorder and improved diagnostic methods can account for increases in prevalence (Fombonne 2005; Fombonne *et al.* 2006). Powell *et al.* (2000) report an incidence of ASD in the general population of approximately eight new cases a year in every 10,000 children and Chakrabarti and Fombonne (2005) recently reported a prevalence of autistic disorder of 22 per 10,000 in children aged four to six years. Fombonne *et al.* (2006) report the same rate of autistic disorder in their survey of more than 27,000 children, with an additional 10 per 10,000 being classified as having Asperger's syndrome. Thus, the incidence in the Jure *et al.* (1991) study of four children in 1000 is very high.

Presentation of ASD in deaf children

Since both deafness and autism affect communication, their co-existence is likely to have severe consequences. Thus, the major problem facing the clinician working with hearing-impaired children is that many of the behaviours described above are apparent in hearing-impaired children to some degree, at some point during their early development. Children with a profound hearing loss, who do not have access to good language models from an early age, are very likely to evidence disordered patterns of communication. This can have a knock-on effect on all aspects of socio-emotional communication, play skills and understanding of and response to others' verbal and non-verbal cues. In addition, deaf children may try to impose structure or order on a world that for them is difficult to make sense of, resulting in restrictive behaviour patterns and the need for predictable routines. However, the fact that these behaviours are so common in hearing-impaired children generally means that there is a real danger of over-diagnosing autism in this group. Conversely, as a result, caution over mis-diagnosing autism in deaf children has led to children who do have genuine autistic-spectrum problems going unrecognized and therefore access to appropriate services is denied (as seen in Jure *et al.* 1991, where 22 per cent of the diagnoses were made very late).

Perhaps the most useful indicators of significant autistic disorder in a deaf child are the absence of communicative intent and behavioural disturbance suggestive of disorder rather than simply delay. In other words, the child must show evidence of a lack of desire to communicate, rather than lack of understandable communication per se. Problems with the development of play skills, joint attention skills, understanding and response to others' emotions, and the need for routine and predictability, must be markedly different from those seen in the general population of hearing-impaired children, for a diagnosis of autistic spectrum disorder to be made. In addition, if the child shows unambiguous evidence of unusual rituals, repetitious behaviour or obsessional interests, these should be taken as strong evidence in support of an ASD diagnosis. As with the diagnosis of any disorder of neuropsychological development, it is important to bear in mind any social and emotional factors that may be affecting the child's responses.

The most useful indicators of significant autistic disorder in a deaf child include the following:

- The absence of communicative intent and behavioural disturbance suggestive of disorder rather than simply delay. In other words, the child must show evidence of a lack of desire to communicate, rather than lack of understandable communication per se.

- Problems with the development of play skills, joint attention skills, understanding and response to others' emotions, and the need for routine and predictability, must be markedly different from those seen in the general population of hearing-impaired children, for a diagnosis of autistic spectrum disorder to be made.

- As with the diagnosis of any disorder of neuropsychological development, it is important to bear in mind any social and emotional factors that may be affecting the child's responses, for example parental depression.

Outcome research

A great number of studies have been conducted examining the impact of a wide variety of interventions for childhood autism. Many of these can be considered psychological, in that they do not involve drugs or dietary modifications. Some of the most frequently researched interventions are those in which the parents of the child carry out the treatment or therapy under the instruction and guidance of psychologists and other therapists – 'parent-mediated interventions'. Unfortunately very few of these can be deemed of good quality in terms of research design or methodology, or fall short of high standards of reporting. Indeed, in a recent Cochrane Review of this literature, Diggle, McConachie and Randle (2007) report that of 68 articles they identified as being relevant, only two studies met the inclusion criteria for the review. They looked for randomized controlled trials with a comparison group, including children aged 1–6:11, using child-related objective outcome measures (language progress, positive behavioural change and parental interaction style) with parents as the primary implementers of the intervention. The majority of the studies were excluded because they had no control group. The two remaining studies, those of Jocelyn *et al.* (1998) and Smith, Groen and Wynn (2000) report some positive effects of parent-mediated early intervention, but conclude that implications for practice cannot be drawn from only two studies where the numbers of participants are small.

Given the lack of robust empirical evidence on the efficacy of interventions in autistic children, it is not surprising that there are no randomized controlled trials of psychological/behavioural interventions for deaf children with ASDs. In fact, we have only been able to locate one report of any sort describing a psychological intervention for an autistic deaf child – a case report. Garcia and Turk (2007) apply the Webster-Stratton Parenting Programmes (see Webster-Stratton 1984) to a ten-year-old deaf boy with Asperger's syndrome. The treatment is intended to involve groups of parents attending a series of 12 sessions covering positive parenting skills, behaviour management skills and providing peer support; however, for a variety of reasons these authors were only able to provide data for one child and his mother. The authors state that the child's mother reported reductions in stress and child problem behaviours, along with improvements in overall behaviour. However, these findings should be considered extremely preliminary given the many methodological inadequacies of the study.

Theoretical perspectives

A number of researchers have proposed theoretical models or made suggestions as to the fundamental or primary deficit in ASD in an attempt to account for the wide range of difficulties and impairments present in autistic disorders. Deficits in language, representational thought and failure to participate in social interaction have each been considered to play a fundamental role, although attempts to establish how the linguistic, cognitive and social deficits may be related to each other have not provided conclusive answers (Shulman, Bukai and Tidhar 2007). Two of the foundations of communication and social skills development have received considerable attention in both autistic and deaf children – theory of mind and communicative intent – and it is to these that we now turn.

Theory of mind

Theory of mind (ToM) is the awareness or understanding that other people may have the same or different intentions, beliefs or desires from our own, and that these mental states influence behaviour. It is often seen as related to an ability to hold shared attention with another person (to the same object or event) and understand meta-representations (Baron-Cohen and Swettenham 1996). Meta-representation is the ability to utilize mental representations of hypothetical events, often seen emerging in children through symbolic play. Having a ToM enables us to put ourself in the position of another, to be able to see a situation from the other's perspective. It is generally felt that these skills emerge in the pre-school years, predominantly through interactions with adults and other children where the child can learn about mental states and how these relate to behaviour (Peterson and Siegal 1995). By four or five years of age, a typically developing child will have a relatively sophisticated understanding of 'false belief' – an awareness that other people can believe something that is not in fact true, and that they will perform an action based on this incorrect belief. In classic ToM experimental tasks, used to assess children's developmental level in this skill, the child is asked to predict what a person (often represented by a puppet or doll) who is unaware of a crucial piece of information believes, for example the location of a hidden object that has been moved in the view of the child but not of the puppet/doll.

ToM development has been extensively researched in autistic children who have consistently been found to be severely delayed in their acquisition of ToM, with many continuing to fail false belief tasks into their teenage years. For example, Happé (1995) reviewed 28 studies with more than 300 autistic participants and concluded that autistic children perform more poorly than age-matched typically developing children even when verbal mental age is taken into account. A meta-analysis of 22 studies that included typically developing controls confirmed this finding (Yirmiya et al. 1998).

There has also been an increasing amount of research in recent years looking at ToM in deaf children not affected by autism, again with generally consistent replication of findings. A number of studies confirm that the performance level of deaf children on ToM tasks is significantly below that of hearing peers and on a par with that of autistic children. For example, in a study by Russell et al. (1998) many children failed false belief questions. Deaf children's performance rose after the age of 13, with the performance of the 8–12-year-olds being no better than the 4–7 year group. Only 14 per cent of the deaf 4–12-year-olds passed the test compared with 85 per cent of 3–5-year-old hearing children. There was still a high failure rate in the 13–16-year group, with 40 per cent not completing the task successfully. However, the issue is complicated in deaf children given the variety of communication modes employed by them, and the efficacy with which they are able to use them. Thus, deaf children of hearing parents who learn to use sign language late (i.e. after the normal period of linguistic development in the toddler years) show very delayed ToM development, whereas deaf children of deaf parents ('native signers') do not demonstrate a deficit (Courtin and Melot 2005; Jackson 2001; Peterson and Siegal 2000: Woolfe, Want and Siegal 2002). Orally trained deaf children, and those with cochlear implants, have been found to have difficulty with ToM tasks comparable with that of the later signing children (e.g. Peterson 2004). Thus, the important factor is not communication mode per se, but rather the linguistic competence of the child. It has also been proposed that ToM ability is dependent on access to conversations about mental states (Moeller and Schick 2006; Peterson and Siegal 1995). Interestingly, Peterson, Wellman and Liu (2005) demonstrated that the stages through which children progress in developing a ToM, whilst delayed in deaf children, are the same as for typically developing hearing children. However, the sequence of steps in autistic children differs after a certain point – understanding of hidden emotion is harder than false belief for hearing, late and native signers, but the reverse is true for autistic children.

The majority of studies in this area have adopted some form of false belief task as the benchmark for inferring the acquisition of a theory of mind. However, Marschark *et al.* (2000) caution that it is unwise to rely on a single measure as an indicator of whether a child has achieved a particular developmental goal. In this instance, understanding of false belief is only one of many aspects of a fully developed ToM that could be assessed. Marschark *et al.* propose that deaf children are equally as proficient as their hearing peers at attributing mental states to others as well as themselves, and provide evidence from a story-telling task to support this contention. They suggest it may be the linguistic complexity of the false belief task, or the fact that children have to predict the behaviour of others based on inferred mental states, rather than simply understand and recognize that mental states lead to behaviour, which poses difficulties for deaf children. Given these findings it is premature to use the concept of ToM to try to differentiate between autistic, deaf and autistic-deaf children.

ASSESSMENT OF THEORY OF MIND

Holding in mind the foregoing discussion, and the fact that some deficits in ToM are not exclusive to autism, assessment of ToM is not a sound basis on which to make a diagnosis of autism in deaf children. However, lack of this ability in the pre-school years and beyond is debilitating for deaf children, and has potentially far-reaching consequences for relationships, emotional development and possibly the ability to live independently as adults. Therefore, it is useful to assess a deaf child's understanding of mental states, in order to guide interventions or rehabilitation. A range of assessments exist in relation to testing theory of mind, but many are language-laden and not standardized on deaf children. Those that may be appropriate, and other approaches include:

- Sally Ann test (see Peterson 2002 for an overview with deaf children)

- Happé stories (requires reading skills or the ability to translate into sign language) (Happé 1994)

- discussions about relationships and reporting of relationship understanding at home and school

- understanding and recognition of emotions (making sure that a deaf child has been exposed to the vocabulary first) (see Baron-Cohen 2003).

Summary of ToM in deaf children

- ToM is acquired at the same time in deaf children of deaf parents as hearing children but significantly delayed in deaf children of hearing parents.

- ToM is related to language development, and thinking (mental representations).

- ToM is *not* related to cognition, emotional disturbance, or language disorder.

- A lack of ToM will have an effect on behaviour, emotions, learning and social relationships.

Communicative intent

Communicative intent, or intentional communication as it is also termed, refers to behaviours that are used with the purpose of eliciting a particular response in another individual. The behaviour involves some degree of social engagement as it is aimed at the listener or recipient, rather than the goal itself. It its broadest sense, communicative intent ranges from pre-verbal gestures such as pointing, through to complete grammatically complex sentences. However, it is the developmentally early forms of intentional communication that are of special interest to us. It is important to distinguish communicative behaviours that are truly intentional and those that elicit something but not intentionally. For example, in a very young infant, crying may communicate hunger or discomfort to a caregiver, but it is unlikely that the baby has planned to elicit this response or understands what the outcome is likely to be. Determining intentionality is not easy (see Shulman *et al.* 2007 for a discussion), but attempts to operationalize it have been made (e.g. Coggins and Carpenter 1981; Wetherby *et al.* 1988). The quality of intentionality in communicative acts can be considered to have three dimensions: the communicative function, for example requesting or declaring/protesting; the form by which intentions are expressed (non-symbolic behaviours, pointing, vocalizations and symbolic communication/words); and use of alternating gaze to direct attention (Shulman *et al.* 2007).

Communicative intent follows a predictable developmental pattern in typically developing children. Intentional communication appears in infants at around nine months of age (e.g. Carpenter, Nagell and Tomasello 1998). At this stage, children begin to use pre-verbal behaviours such as gestures and vocalizations to elicit a response from the person they are interacting with. Around 12 to 18 months, when language is developing, children begin to communicate intentionally with words (or signs) with an increasing degree of complexity.

One of the first indications that a child's communication development is deviating from the typical trajectory is when they fail to show normal use of intentional communication. An autistic child who communicates through gestures and vocalization may use these in an idiosyncratic, unusual manner, leaving the observer unsure what the child is trying to convey. Research has shown that young autistic children perform as many communicative acts as typically developing children matched for language level (Prizant and Schuler 1997) but that these acts are more limited in terms of their communicative functions and means.

At around the same time as communicative intent appears in infancy, the related function of joint attention also emerges. Joint attention occurs when a child uses gaze and/or pointing to direct another person's attention to a third object, so that they have a shared understanding regarding the focus of their communication. Joint attention skills have also been found to be atypical or absent in autistic children (Mundy, Sigman and Kasari 1994) and are related to problems in accompanying communication with appropriate use of gaze. Shulman *et al.* (2007, p.129) argue that 'communicative intent has emerged as a pivotal issue in the study of autism. In addition to having implications for intervention, communicative intent may provide a standard of reference from which children with autism can be differentiated from one another', and also, therefore, from other groups of non-autistic children.

In deaf children, joint attention usually begins to appear at around 12 months of age, in line with their hearing peers (Spencer 2000). Similarly, deaf children of hearing parents communicate intentionally with equal frequency as their hearing counterparts at 12, 18 and 22 months of age (Lederberg and

Everhart 1998). However, the nature of the vocalizations differ in terms of the range of sounds used and after around 18 months of age, hearing children progress from primarily non-linguistic communication to linguistic communication, whereas deaf children of hearing parents do not. At about this time, these groups also start to diverge in terms of the amount and nature of joint attention (e.g. Prezbindowski, Adamson and Lederberg 1998), with hearing children increasingly engaging in symbolic joint attention using language, rather than joint attention relating to concrete objects. Deaf children of hearing parents are more likely to use communication to direct or request than to comment or ask questions.

The relevance of these empirical observations to the assessment of ASD in deaf children lies in the differing presentations of communicative intent in autistic children and non-autistic deaf children, and the development of joint attention. Although deaf children do not demonstrate entirely normal skills in this area, particularly after the age of around two years, they do develop pre-verbal communicative intent and joint attention skills, which autistic children typically do not. Therefore, assessment of a deaf child's communicative intent can be very informative as part of a comprehensive assessment of social communication difficulties or ASD.

In a deaf child, communicative intent will be observed by the way a child tries to communicate with another person even if they have a poor range of skills with which to do so. A typically developing deaf child will attempt to communicate and engage with whatever skill they have, even if they have trouble making themselves understood. Even small babies and children with severe learning disabilities in addition to their deafness, usually try to engage and communicate regardless of their skill level. An absence of intent to communicate is even more apparent in a child whose non-verbal cognitive abilities are in the average range. Thus, a deaf child would be expected to want to communicate in any way possible, even if they have not been exposed to accessible language models. However, since the absence of communicative intent is not only present in communication disorders, it is always necessary for the clinician to take a thorough history and to have excluded the possibility of other causes of problems in this area, for example parental depression or abuse, which might be underlying withdrawal behaviour in a child.

ASSESSMENT OF COMMUNICATIVE INTENT

In an assessment of communicative intent, the clinician will formulate the presence or absence of communicative intent through the observation of, and interaction with, the child, along with information from caregivers, looking for the following indicators:

- A general sense of engagement with familiar as well as unfamiliar people, adults and children.

- A sense that the child knows that you are there.

- The child's ability to express pleasure as well as their needs.

- Non-verbal communication on tasks or activities other than highly motivating ones (for example when food is present and desired).

- A desire to communicate with another person, regardless of language skills.

- Joint attention skills, for example sharing a simple picture book where the child points to a picture and looks at the face of the adult, then back at the picture.

- Absence of indications of maternal depression and unavailability or neglect or other forms of abuse.

Assessment and diagnosis of autistic spectrum disorders

DSM-IV (American Psychiatric Association 1994) or *ICD-10* (World Health Organization 1992) classifications should be followed when assessing for autism, both in relation to terminology and diagnosis. A number of additional sources have been developed over recent years that provide guidelines on best practice in assessing and diagnosing ASDs, and also in some cases in terms of intervention.

In all cases of assessment for autism, following national guidelines for gold standard procedures is essential whether a child has known additional difficulties (i.e. deafness) or not. The following texts are available to aid psychologists and child mental health services in providing appropriate services:

- National Initiative for Autism: Screening and Assessment (2003) *National Autism Plan for Children* (*NAPC*) National Autistic Society

- Department of Health (2004) *National Service Framework (NSF) for Children, Young People and Maternity Services* Autism Exemplar

- Department of Health (2003) *Every Child Matters*

- British Psychological Society (2006a) *Autistic Spectrum Disorders: Guidance for Chartered Psychologists Working with Children and Young People*

The NAPC (see above) identifies the following five stages to assessment:

1. *Identification*: for example training of all professionals in 'alerting' signals of possible ASD; surveillance; local audit of ASD detection and diagnosis.

2. *Assessment*:
    Stage 1 – General Developmental Assessment, notification to education
    Stage 2 – Multi-agency Assessment (ten essential components outlined), locality-based, named key worker, assessment completed and feedback given within 17 weeks of Stage 2
    Stage 3 – referral on to tertiary ASD assessment (e.g. second opinion).

3. *Interventions*: within six weeks of the end of Assessment Stage 2, information provided, intervention specific for ASD.

4. *Resources*: recommended services should be jointly commissioned (e.g. key workers), local strategic planning and dissemination.

5. *Training*: multi-agency awareness training, evaluation and audit.

Assessment in deaf children

Assessment of autism in deaf children is complicated and the diagnosis is diffi-cult to make due to the complex interplay of neurological deficits, communica-tion modes and styles as well as the typical delay in language acquisition in deaf children. It is therefore essential that the assessment is made involving a team of varying professionals (multi-disciplinary team (MDT)), ideally including those who have an understanding of deafness. Ideally, the MDT should consist of a speech and language therapist specializing in deafness, child psychiatrist and clinical psychologist. An occupational therapist and paediatrician can be a useful part of the assessment where a differential diagnosis is needed. Links to local services including education and educational psychology are essential. The opportunity to see children across time is useful as the rate of developmen-tal change can be monitored, and seeing children established in an educational setting can be beneficial for observation of the child in structured and peer settings, and also to see their learning potential.

ASSESSMENT SCHEDULES AND QUESTIONNAIRES

A number of assessment schedules and questionnaires are available, which can help guide diagnosis. Some are more useful than others in the hearing-impaired population. The Autism Diagnostic Observation Schedule-Generic (ADOS-G; Lord *et al.* 2000) is a standardized, interactive schedule based on a series of structured and semi-structured situations, in which the behavioural responses of the child are rated. The schedule is appropriate for children with no expressive language, through to verbally fluent, high-functioning adolescents and adults. However, even in the youngest children, some understanding of what the examiner is asking the child to do is required, and several of the items to be rated are directly dependent on the child's verbal communication skills. The ADOS-G has been shown to have good validity, reliability and diagnostic utility, but as yet there are no studies specifically investigating its use in the hearing-impaired population.

A range of questionnaires is also available to aid in the assessment of autism, for example the Autism Diagnostic Interview – Revised (Lord, Rutter and LeCouteur 1994) but are not standardized on a hearing-impaired population. Unfortunately, they do not clearly differentiate behaviours that could be attributable to either deafness or autism. Thus, great care must be taken when interpreting the results and a sound knowledge of the 'normal' communication and behaviour patterns of hearing-impaired children is essential.

As with all deaf children where there is a suspected communication disorder, a non-verbal cognitive assessment is essential (see Chapter 4 for more information on this). Play-based assessment (Linder 1993) can be used in addition to cognitive assessment, or instead of cognitive assessment for children who are younger than two years old, or for those whose skills prevent them from completing a formal assessment tool.

An assessment to find out whether learning difficulties are also present is essential. Meeting the needs of a child affected by deafness and autism will take a lot of expertise. Profiling all of their needs and not just the deafness is paramount. Sometimes the deafness is not the primary disability as may be seen from the following case example, and thus considering an appropriate educational placement may need to reflect this.

Case example: Assessing more than deafness

George, aged three years, was born overseas. He has a bilateral profound sensori-neural hearing loss. He lives at home with his parents and older brother (who has a moderate hearing loss). He attends a mainstream pre-school playgroup each morning and receives support from a local teacher of the deaf, a speech and language therapist and an educational psychologist. English is not the family's first language, but the family use English, without an interpreter (at their request) during assessment appointments. George's father works, and his mother is at home. Mother's family live overseas.

George was not referred regarding concerns about his social communication, but for an assessment for cochlear implantation. During this assessment the team became concerned about whether George had emotional
difficulties, relating to family history or whether he had a social communication disorder.

The assessment was carried out by an audiological scientist, a consultant
in audiological medicine, a specialist speech and language therapist and a
clinical psychologist. Links were made to social services, the pre-school
special educational needs coordinator, educational psychologist, and local
teacher of the deaf and speech and language therapist, for further information. The assessment was completed in sign language, which George had only
begun to learn recently.

Clinical psychology assessment process

- Assessment at school and in the clinic over three months.

- Video recordings of George playing at home with his mother were
  viewed.

- A play-based assessment was completed.

- Non-verbal cognitive abilities assessment was completed (SON-R;
  Snijders *et al.* 1989; Tellegen *et al.* 1998).

- *DSM-IV* diagnostic criteria were employed.

ASSESSMENT FINDINGS
Development and cognitive abilities, from parental report, school observation and formal assessment

- George was described as a quiet baby.

- George was toilet trained age two-and-a-half and is currently dry day
  and night.

- George completed a ten-piece inset puzzle independently. He looked
  at books and was able to match a toy animal with a picture when
  modelled first.

- George was able to begin to copy a line and circle. He enjoyed line
  and circular scribble and was very particular about the pencils that he
  chose, putting them back in the correct colour pots.

- George tidied up items only when given explicit instructions to do so. He was unable to generalize this and tidy up in other contexts.

- At snack time at school, he gave the cups out when instructed.

- George scored in the average range on the SON-R, however it was difficult for him to follow adult-led tasks, and required a lot of prompting to complete four of the six sub-tests.

Social interaction and communicative intent

- George was not observed to show communicative intent other than to share pleasure on one occasion when pushing bricks down a slide in a clinic session.

- He did not approach an adult or his parents to play in the clinic.

- When adult-led interaction finished (even high-interest games), he did not attempt to resume games; he would just sit and stare.

- When an adult sat next to him at school whilst he was drawing, it was many minutes before he noticed that someone was sitting there. Once he noticed, he stared.

- No facial expressions were seen, other than smiling at the end of the session with his parents.

- No interaction with the other children at school was observed, however he was happy to play alongside them.

- George follows nursery routines. He watches the other children in order to know what he is expected to do.

- George was observed not to join in with action songs at school, and was unable to access the story time due to lack of signing by the teachers. At these times he would look around him at any movement in the room.

Communication

- George signed 'toilet' after a model from his mother.

- He was very independent, for example he tried several times to fit a ramp on to a toy. Even with clear indications that an adult could help him, he did not request support. Eventually he moved the item towards the adult, and pulled their hand requesting help (using their hand as a tool).

- It was very difficult to obtain George's eye contact, even with physical prompting, and being on the same level and facing him.

- George's pre-verbal skills were poor, with limited referential looking, and no referential pointing seen. He was able to point between two similar items, but without eye contact to an adult.

- No spontaneous turn-taking was established after many attempts. An adult was able to intrude and take a turn only if they 'jumped' in.

- George was observed to be very passive; if someone blocked his path, then he would go around them rather than communicate with the person to move.

- In the play house at school, George vocalized briefly using open vowel sounds. This was the only time that he was observed to vocalize at school.

- No spontaneous signs were seen at clinic or in school.

Play

- George was very passive in play, using only the items that he was handed. He did not explore all the toys available to him.

- George predominantly enjoyed a repetitive game of pushing cars down a ramp. At home he is described as mainly playing with cars whilst lying on the floor.

- He did not purposefully move his play on without an adult's model first, for example catching cars in a pan. He would then take on this idea, but again was unable to develop it further unless shown.

- An adult was able to intrude in George's play.

- George demonstrated relational play with a doll and household items.

- In the playground, George enjoyed using pedal cars. He particularly liked parking the cars at the end of the session. He gestured at the end of the play session to the children to come away from the cars, so that he could park them all neatly.

- In the play house in the playground, where two other children were already playing, he did not interact with them, but played his own game.

- George's play often included organizing items.

Behaviour

- George's parents report that at home George requires a certain bottle to be filled to the top with milk, even though he always only drinks half. He has fixed routines, for example he insists on being the first in and out of the door at home, and he has to be the first into the car. If this is not the case, then the family have to start the routine again.

- George is very aware of routines at home, for example gets a change of clothes for his brother when it is time to pick up his brother from school.

- George is reportedly very tidy, with items having to go back in certain places.

- George is described as independent, for example helping himself to food from the fridge.

- There is a possibility that George hyperventilates at times, as he was observed to yawn a lot during times of transition between activities. This may be due to anxiety about what is expected of him and uncertainty about what is happening next. He also appears to be hypervigilant, staring with reduced blinking, possibly for the same reasons as the hyperventilation.

Family issues

- George and his mother remained overseas while his father came to the UK. He and his family joined his father here just before he was two.

- His mother would like to return home, and appears mildly depressed. She has no family in the UK; the father's family is here.

DSM-IV criteria

1. *Qualitative impairment in social interaction in two areas:* George met criteria for lack of use of multiple non-verbal behaviours – failure to develop peer relationships appropriate to developmental level, and a lack of spontaneous seeking to share pleasure.

2. *Qualitative impairments in communication in at least one area:* George did not meet criteria for delay or lack of development of spoken language because of his deafness, and it was difficult to judge his development in sign language as he was late beginning to learn (at approximately three years of age). Similarly, it was difficult to assess him on his ability to start or sustain conversations. His use of stereotyped or repetitive language could not be assessed due to the absence of language. Finally, he met criteria for lack of sponta-neous make-believe play. However, caution must be exercised here as make-believe play is linked to language development.

3. *Restrictive repetitive and stereotyped patterns of behaviour:* George did not show preoccupations with parts of objects, or demonstrate motor mannerisms. He did meet criteria for adherence to non-functional routines, but not with restrictive patterns of interests. Again, we need to be cautious here as a deaf child without useful language is going to rely on routines to understand his world.

ASSESSMENT CONCLUSIONS IN RELATION TO COMMUNICATION DISORDER

Overall, George's cognitive skills appear age-appropriate, with his social com-munication delayed to that of a one-year-old child. His pre-verbal skills are sig-nificantly delayed and disordered, which will affect his ability to communicate with others, regardless of how accomplished he becomes in his signing skills. His communicative intent is delayed regardless of his delay in being taught to use sign. This will have secondary effects on his learning and thus needs to be addressed in conjunction with his deafness. His passivity may also be linked to low mood, however this was difficult to assess. In relation to autism, George did meet the *DSM-IV* criteria, however caution was advised due to his family circumstances, possible maternal depression and significant language needs. A diagnosis of social communication disorder was therefore made, with a recommendation of reviewing and reassessing him after one year to see how his language skills had progressed, and to see if this had an impact on the areas of functioning that were currently atypical.

Conclusions

In this chapter we have focused primarily on the practical issues of assessing deaf children who present with social communication difficulties. Our aim has been to clarify the distinction between various types of communication difficulties and their presentation in deaf children, and to provide suggestions regarding assessment strategies. As the case example illustrates, this can be a complex process requiring a skilled team of professionals with understanding of deafness as well as communication and autism spectrum disorders. The paucity of tools to aid diagnosis in deaf children as well as lack of research does not help clinicians to feel secure in their practice. Caution must be exercised when making a diagnosis where clinical features can be present for a number of reasons, but equally, deaf children should not be prevented from having specialist assessments just because they are deaf; attributing all of their needs to deafness will result in serious consequences for their education, social skills, peer relationships and ultimately mental health.

6 Paediatric Cochlear Implantation

Cochlear implants can provide children who have a severe to profound sensori-neural hearing loss with a sensation of hearing, which in a significant proportion of children can lead to normal or near normal oral language development. At the time of writing this chapter, the majority of children who may benefit from a cochlear implant receive a single (rather than bilateral) implant, giving them uni-directional access to sound. Some continue to use a hearing aid in the other ear, if they gain some useful hearing from it. Although cochlear implants may transform the lives of many deaf children (and hence arguably that of their families too), implants are not without controversy. Concerns have been raised by the Deaf community, both here in the UK and in the USA, and other countries, that cochlear implants will result in the demise of Deaf culture, including the use of signed languages such as BSL, ASL and Auslan. However, given that 90 per cent of deaf children are born to hearing parents and that cochlear implants have been found to be a safe, effective means of providing auditory stimulation, it is not surprising that in the UK alone around 250 children receive cochlear implants each year. Cochlear implantation is one of the few interventions used with deaf children where there is a very large empirical research base on outcomes in terms of speech perception, speech intelligibility, language and communication skills. Psychological, educational and social outcomes have received considerably less attention, but there is a growing literature in these areas.

In this chapter we will consider the role of psychologists in the field of cochlear implants, with particular emphasis on the psychological assessment of children before implantation. We will consider the issue of consent to treatment in children and adolescents for whom a cochlear implant is recommended, and describe the type of psychological input that may be required in the months and years after the child has received an implant.

Why cochlear implants and clinical psychology?

Paediatric Cochlear Implant Programmes are multi-disciplinary. They typically comprise audiologists, speech and language therapists, teachers of the deaf, ENT surgeons and audiological physicians. Some also include clinical psychologists and hearing therapists, although these are relatively few and far between. Most Paediatric Cochlear Implant Programmes use a 'consultancy' model for psychological input for the children, 'buying in' psychological services when a specific need has been identified, for example where there is a query regarding a child's developmental status or there are behavioural problems that will impede progress following implantation. In contrast, we strongly advocate a model of working where clinical psychologists are an integral, permanent part of the multi-disciplinary team. There are a number of reasons for this, summarized below:

- The threshold for referral to psychology is probably lower, more appropriate and prevents escalation of problems.

- Problems can be dealt with more quickly and effectively.

- Parents cannot 'opt out' of psychology, as it is part of the package of care.

- The psychologist can more quickly gain the specialist experience and expertise needed to work with deaf children, which improves patient care.

- Liaison with other team members is more efficient.

- Psychology is perceived by the families as a normal part of the service and is therefore less potentially stigmatizing.

- The psychologist can obtain systematic baseline measures of cognition or development.

The potential role of clinical psychologists within the multi-disciplinary team is varied and far-reaching. Although psychologists were not historically part of Paediatric Cochlear Implant Programme teams, where they have become established as such they provide a specialist service, including assessment, individual, family and group interventions and liaison with local health, educational and social services.

Clinical psychologists may be involved with children at any stage of the programme – from pre-implant assessment, preparation for surgery and switch-on to post-implant follow-up. Their input is also likely to be indicated in cases where children or adolescents are at risk of becoming non-users, that is, stopping use of the device against the advice of the professionals involved in their care and against the wishes of their family. Each of these areas will be explored fully in later sections following the path children and their families take on a typical Cochlear Implant Programme.

Research

Paediatric cochlear implantation is one of the few areas within the field of deafness where there is a very substantial outcome literature base, although perhaps surprisingly, as yet there has been no Cochrane Review, and National Institute for Clinical Excellence (NICE) guidelines on good practice are due to be available during 2008. Much of the research in this area uses a cross-sectional design, where children with cochlear implants are compared with age or language-level matched hearing children, or with deaf children without cochlear implants. Other studies employ a longitudinal, cohort design where the progress of a group of children is monitored over time. The quality of studies varies considerably, in terms of the homogeneity of groups, the extent to which partic-ipants are 'matched' between groups (on variables such as pre-implant language abilities, additional disabilities, educational placement, communication mode) and so on. Unfortunately the literature is so large, and varied in its focus, it is not possible to give more than a flavour of the area here.

Cochlear implants are able to give a consistent auditory signal for all the sounds that make up speech, and a level of loudness that is very similar in all recipients. However, despite this consistency, the degree of benefit individual children derive from their implant varies enormously, with some children achieving oral language skills that are as good as their hearing peers, whilst others develop very limited oral language and their speech intelligibility is poor. Readers interested in the outcome literature for paediatric cochlear implants may like to consult Thoutenhoofd et al. (2005), who provide a critical review of all the relevant papers published between 1994 and 2001.

A number of factors have consistently been found to be predictive of good speech and language outcomes, the most reliable of which is the age at which the child receives his or her implant, with earlier implantation associated with the best results (e.g. Connor et al. 2006; McConkey Robbins et al. 2004). Other significant variables include the length of time the child has been severely/

profoundly deaf (in the case of progressive, sudden or post-lingual deafness) and the type of educational approach employed (e.g. signed, oral or Total Communication). Geers (2006) provides a review of factors influencing outcomes in children who have had a cochlear implant at a young age. It is increasingly becoming apparent that a number of psychosocial issues are also of relevance, although there continues to be relatively little research from this perspective. A handful of papers have been published in each of the following areas: parental stress, behaviour, quality of life, self-concept/self-esteem and developmental delay. A slightly more substantial literature exists on the relevance of cognitive factors in paediatric cochlear implantation (e.g. Khan, Edwards and Langdon 2005; Shin *et al.* 2007; Surowiecki *et al.* 2002).

Of note in terms of the role of clinical psychologists on Cochlear Implant Programme teams is research examining the impact of implantation for children with complex needs, or those with difficulties in addition to their deafness, which is reviewed by Edwards (2007). Most paediatric cochlear implant research only reports outcomes from children with no disabilities in addition to their deafness. A few reports of outcomes exist for children with additional difficulties, and by and large, these suggest more limited benefit in terms of speech and language although quality of life, if assessed, is generally thought to be enhanced. Findings such as these emphasize the need for thorough psychological assessment of cochlear implant candidates, encompassing areas such as general development, cognitive abilities, social communication skills, parental (and, where possible, child) expectations and quality of life.

Assessment for paediatric cochlear implantation

Where the psychologist is a permanent, integral member of the Cochlear Implant Programme team, a significant aspect of the role is the assessment of deaf children being considered for cochlear implantation. A comprehensive assessment involves both the child and his or her family and is likely to require at least two sessions to complete. In complex cases the process may take considerably longer with multiple sessions over a period of several weeks or even months. However, given the importance of implanting children as young as possible for the best outcomes, the assessment should be completed in as timely a fashion as possible. It is also important to remember that the psychological assessment takes place in the context of a number of assessments by the other members of the cochlear implant team, and families can feel quite overwhelmed by the number of appointments, especially if there are siblings whose needs must also not be forgotten. Although it may sometimes appear that a child and his or her family are 'straightforward' in terms of the appropriateness of a cochlear implant for the child, and therefore a psychological assessment may seem unnecessary, we believe that it is essential that all children who are being considered for an implant be assessed as routine.

Rationale for psychological assessment

There are a number of reasons why a psychological assessment is useful pre-implantation. One of the main purposes is to identify any issues or areas of difficulty that may influence how the child and his or her family adapt to the implant. This may be in terms of the child's learning style or cognitive abilities, their behaviour or emotional state, their prior use of hearing aids, or the family's attitude towards deafness, their understanding of what a cochlear implant can offer or local support they have access to. Other issues may include parental mental health and the relationship between the deaf child and his or her siblings. It is important to identify any significant difficulties as early as possible, so that where possible, appropriate intervention or support can be offered before the child receives the implant. It is not unusual for the psychological assessment to highlight developmental or learning problems that have not previously been documented, and where this is the case, such difficulties may have an impact on the potential benefit the child can receive from an implant. Therefore, a second important function of the psychological assessment is to gain information that can help parents make an informed choice regarding whether or not they wish their child to proceed with implantation. Counselling parents, and, where appropriate, the child or adolescent, about likely outcomes, particularly where the child has multiple disabilities or complex needs, can be a lengthy process as the issues are often very complicated and families often have high hopes and expectations about what an implant can offer.

The next reason for completing a psychological assessment is to collect 'baseline' information against which future progress can be compared. Again, particularly where there are significant developmental, learning or behavioural issues, these need to be monitored and input offered as required. Finally, as mentioned previously, the psychological assessment forms part of a comprehensive, multi-disciplinary assessment and therefore the results of the psychological assessment need to be considered within this context. When all the information from the assessments is considered together, some inconsistencies or discrepancies may be revealed that are of significance in terms of the child's suitability for implantation. A possible scenario is given in the case example below.

When meeting families for the first time it is useful to be able to give them a rationale for the psychological assessment. It can be explained that all children are seen by a psychologist so that a picture of the 'whole child' can be obtained, including an understanding of their personality, temperament, likes and dislikes, so that the cochlear implant process can be tailored to them as an

> **Case example: Multi-disciplinary findings of pre-implant assessment**
>
> - Boy aged four years six months, diagnosed hearing-impaired aged eight months, aided aged ten months, some access to speech sounds in the lower frequencies.
> - Sign language used within the home since around one year of age, and in nursery from three years of age.
> - Above-average non-verbal cognitive abilities.
> - Functionally, the child shows very little awareness of environmental sounds, is using only single signs, and producing no speech sounds, even those to which he has access auditorily.
>
> These findings are not what would be expected in a typically developing deaf child. Given his good cognitive abilities, the length of time he has been exposed to signed communication and his access to sounds (including speech) in the lower frequencies, we would predict that this child should be responding to some environmental sounds, using some vocalizations approximating the speech sounds he is able to detect, and putting at least three to four signs together to make sentences. The fact that he appears to be making little use of the residual hearing that he has, and that he is not making appropriate progress in developing language skills using sign, cannot be accounted for by a generalized learning problem. Therefore, it is possible that this little boy has a specific language difficulty, which is interfering with both his spoken and sign language development, and this would need to be investigated further before a decision about cochlear implantation could be made.

individual, as far as this is practicable. This can allay parents' fears that they have been 'selected' in some way to see a psychologist, because there is something 'wrong' with them or their child. It is also helpful to explain that the results of the assessment will provide useful information about the potential benefit the child may receive from an implant, to aid the parents (and possibly child) in decision-making regarding proceeding with an implant.

Assessment of family issues
TIME OF DIAGNOSIS OF DEAFNESS

One of the first areas to explore with parents is their experience of the time of diagnosis of deafness. As we saw in Chapter 1, some very strong emotions are typically engendered around this time, and it is not uncommon for parents to have unresolved issues, even some years later. Parents have sometimes not previously had the opportunity to discuss issues around diagnosis and their understanding of deafness and its impact, so may find it helpful to consider these with someone who was not involved in the child's care at that time.

Although Newborn Hearing Screening Programmes are identifying hearing-impairment in children at a much younger age than previously, some children are still not being referred for cochlear implantation until they are two or even three years old. This may be for a number of reasons, including parental choice, so it is important to ask the question 'Why now?' in terms of seeking an implant for their child. It may be that they were advised or wanted to 'wait and see' whether their child would develop oral communication with his or her hearing aids, and then realized that they were not making adequate progress. Alternatively, the diagnosis of hearing-impairment may have been delayed, leaving parents with a sense that time has been wasted or lost, and feelings of anger or depression.

ACCEPTANCE OF DEAFNESS

Parents' understanding and acceptance of any additional difficulties their child may be known to have is an important area to explore. Where deafness is part of a syndrome, with significant other medical, physical or learning problems, the impact of a cochlear implant on the child's capacity to develop oral communication skills may be relatively limited. It is often hard for parents not to see a cochlear implant as in some way resolving many of the other problems a multiply disabled child faces. There is often a link between the parents' acceptance of their child's deafness, and the child's use of hearing aids, particularly in young children. Although many pre-school children do not wear their hearing aids consistently for behavioural reasons, in a significant proportion, non-use is rooted in parental denial of the hearing-impairment, a desire to hide the disability, or feelings of guilt if the deafness has a genetic aetiology.

USE OF HEARING AIDS

A substantial amount of time frequently needs to be given to discussing hearing aid use. Compliance with wearing hearing aids is usually a good predictor of the child's acceptance of the implant device, so it is crucial that any problems with wearing them are resolved well before a child receives a cochlear implant. In some cases, as described above, non-compliance may be associated with emotional issues in the parents, but more often it is simply the result of lack of firm encouragement to wear them on the part of the parents. In toddlers, non-compliance is typically part of a picture of difficult behaviours, and a realization that pulling them out every few minutes is guaranteed to get lots of parental attention! Sometimes parents are unaware of the importance of their child wearing the aids, especially if they appear to receive limited benefit, and once this is explained, parents usually quickly enforce an appropriate regime of hearing aid use. Where compliance remains poor it is usual for the psychologist to offer intervention sessions to address this, as non-use can prevent the other members of the team from being able to carry out their assessments. Very occasionally, poor compliance with wearing hearing aids is associated with pain or discomfort, hyperacusis, tinnitus or phonophobia, or self-image issues in older children. These also need addressing appropriately, and may require input from a range of professionals.

COMMUNICATION ISSUES

Other areas to include when talking to the parents are their understanding of the child's communication needs and the impact of their deafness on the educational provision they will require. Attitudes towards discipline and boundary-setting, coping styles and strategies when faced with difficulties and access to social and professional support are all areas that are highly relevant to explore. Occasionally there are issues around parental mental health that are having a significant impact on parental insight and coping, and these should be addressed when necessary. The roles of culture and religion in relation to disability are important factors to consider in all families, as are views regarding the place of Deaf culture and BSL for any individual child and family.

EXPECTATIONS

Hopes and expectations surround the process of cochlear implantation and have implications for perceptions of satisfaction throughout the process from pre-implant to long-term follow-up. Where expectations are realistic they are likely to contribute to optimizing outcome. A clear understanding and acceptance of the potential benefits and limitations of a cochlear implant, in comparison with alternative options, helps parents to make an informed choice. Parents can be helped to arrive at realistic expectations through the use of video material and contact with other parents of children with implants, reflecting a range of experiences, both positive and negative. It can also be useful for parents to meet others who have decided not to go ahead with an implant for their child, to explore the alternatives in terms of communication mode and educational provision.

SIBLINGS

It is not uncommon for more than one child within a family to have a hearing loss and be assessed for cochlear implantation. However, siblings do not necessarily have the same degree of hearing loss, or they may differ markedly in terms of the additional difficulties they have. Therefore, a cochlear implant may be considered likely to benefit one child but not his or her brother or sister, resulting in differences in the types of hearing devices used by them and possibly in the choice of communication modes and schools for them. This is likely to have both practical and psychological implications for the children and their parents that need to be carefully considered as part of the assessment process.

The siblings of a child who is undergoing cochlear implant assessment may have fears about some of the tests and investigations their brother or sister is having, or be scared about them having an operation. Including siblings in the assessment process ensures that these issues are addressed when needed, and can prevent problems occurring later on.

The areas to explore with parents, and, where appropriate, siblings, during the psychological assessment are summarized below:

- history of the diagnosis of deafness and course of hearing loss (if not stable)

- understanding and acceptance of additional difficulties

- parental coping strategies and access to social and professional support

- parental mental health and family functioning

- communication choices

- hearing aid compliance

- parenting style, including bonding and setting boundaries

- culture and religion

- expectations.

Developmental assessment

The general development of deaf children in areas other than their speech, language and communication, is an important indicator of the child's learning capacity and therefore a useful predictor of their use of the implant and the progress they should make with it. An understanding of the child's general development is also useful in terms of tailoring the assessment process and post-implant (re)habilitation to the specific needs of that child. Clearly, as the child gets older, information regarding their very early development may become less relevant, particularly in adolescents, but some early factors may continue to play a role in the child's development well into the primary school years. In very young children, particularly those under two years of age, it is not possible to gain a non-verbal IQ estimate using standard psychometric tests, even those intended for use in children with limited language skills. Where possible in children over two years it is preferable to administer a non-verbal assessment of cognitive abilities – see the next section for further details. Many children aged from two to around three years are unable to tackle formal cognitive tests for a variety of reasons – temperament, behaviour, attention and concentration, and of course as a result of developmental delay, placing their cognitive abilities below the floor for the test, or social communication difficulties. Thus, in this group, and for those under two years of age, it is useful to administer a standardized developmental assessment such as the Griffiths Mental Development Scales (Griffiths 1984), the Bayley Scales of Infant and Toddler Development (Bayley 2005) or the Schedule of Growing Skills II (Bellman, Lingham and Aukett 1996). However, only those sections or sub-tests that do not assess the development of speech, language or communication should be attempted, as the results of those would be invalid due to the child's deafness. Also, the speech and language therapists on the team will undertake a comprehensive, detailed assessment of these areas, making the limited information to be gained from a typical developmental assessment redundant.

The skill domains covered by these developmental assessments are very similar, and generally include areas such as gross and fine motor skills, visual-perceptual abilities, personal-social and interactive skills, and, usually inferred from other abilities, cognitive abilities. These assessments are based on a combination of information from a parent or primary caregiver, and direct observation of the child's abilities. Even with very young children it is usually possible to convey the requirements of a task, through the use of demonstration, gesture, repetition and a lot of patience!

Assessment of cognitive abilities and learning style

The assessment of paediatric cochlear implant candidates' cognitive abilities could be considered one of the most important aspects of the psychological assessment, for reasons that have been discussed earlier. One of the main purposes of the cognitive assessment is to establish whether the child has global learning difficulties or any specific difficulties that may impact on his or her ability to learn to understand the auditory input provided by a cochlear implant. Where such difficulties are identified, this may not have been anticipated by the parents and therefore the information may come as a shock, or be greeted with anger or distress. The implications of the results of the cognitive assessment need to be carefully explained to the child's parents, and indeed to the local professionals working with the child, so that expectations are realistic and interventions can be tailored to the specific needs and capabilities of the child. It is advisable to contact the child's educational psychologist if they have one, to see whether they have already undergone cognitive testing, as most assessments should not be repeatedly administered without a suitable time lapse in between.

There are only two commonly used tests that are suitable for deaf children: the Leiter International Performance Scale – Revised (Leiter-R; Roid and Miller 1997), and the Snijders-Oomen Non-verbal Intellectual Test (SON-R; Snijders *et al.* 1989; Tellegen *et al.* 1998). Both provide an overall non-verbal IQ estimate based on a series of sub-scales. The range of cognitive abilities covered by the tests is greater in the Leiter-R, and this test also has the advantage of allowing the child's visual memory and attention abilities to be assessed. It also has the advantage that it covers a very wide age range, from 2:0 to 20:11, and children generally appear to enjoy the tasks since they are visually appealing and allow him or her to experience success with ease in the early test items. However, in the youngest children for whom the test can be used (and those at the upper end of the age range) the norms for the Leiter-R are somewhat problematic since the full range of scaled scores is not used on some sub-tests; in older children and young adults some scaled scores are not provided at the upper end of the ability range and in very young children they are not available at the bottom of the range, leading to poor discrimination of degree of learning disability.

Related to a child's cognitive abilities is their learning style, or the way in which they tackle novel tasks and make use of feedback and contextual information. Many deaf children are somewhat rigid or inflexible in the way they approach activities or tests, having difficulty altering the way they respond to changes in the nature of the task or in response to feedback about their performance. For example, they may continue to match stimuli based on colour when the task has changed to one of working out a sequence based on size. The child's learning style is best assessed by close observation of the way in which they tackle the developmental assessment or non-verbal cognitive assessment, along with observation of the way they respond to adult-directed activities in general. It can also include observation of their interactions with an adult who is trying to engage them in play in a particular way, giving information about their social communication skills.

Learning style has implications for the way in which a child adapts to the new auditory stimulation provided by a cochlear implant, along with how they cope with the activities of rehabilitation suggested by the Cochlear Implant Programme team teachers and/or speech and language therapists.

Assessment of play

As with the psychological assessment of children in other fields, for example in child and adolescent mental health services or child development services, the assessment of play skills is an important part of the cochlear implant assessment. In hearing-impaired children, assessment of play can be particularly informative especially where a formal cognitive developmental assessment is not possible, perhaps as a result of temperament, cooperation or significant additional difficulties. Play skills typically follow a well-defined, predictable developmental sequence and therefore produce an invaluable, if rough, guide to the child's developmental level. Play assessment can be approached either formally using an instrument such as the Symbolic Play Test (Lowe and Costello 1995), or informally by observing play in a clinic, the home or educational setting. Often the most information is gained from the latter approach, especially if it is possible to visit the child at home or nursery as part of the cochlear implant assessment process.

A number of aspects of the child's play should be considered. In the youngest children the psychologist can look for evidence of joint attention skills and the ability to take turns in play. Different types of play such as exploratory (mouthing, touch), relational, pretend, symbolic and imaginary play should be noted, as should evidence of the ability to match and sort (e.g. colour, shape, size), label objects or problem-solve. The child can be encouraged to use a pencil or crayon on paper, noting whether they produce to-and-fro or circular scribbles, or can copy simple lines or shapes (circle, cross etc.). In slightly older children, up to around four years of age, it is useful to observe the range and types of toys explored, for example whether they are concrete (construction toys or puzzles), or whether there is a preference for activities such as dressing up, pretend play with dolls, or symbolic play with cars, trains, dolls house and so on.

Whilst assessing the child's play skills it is also useful to observe other aspects of their behaviour. For example, their attention and concentration skills should be noted along with how the child reacts to someone else (the assessor, parent or sibling) joining in their play. The child's ability to incorporate another person in their play, adapt what they are doing and include others' ideas, are important in terms of understanding the child's level of social and emotional development.

If the hearing-impaired child appears not to be developing typical play skills for his or her age it is important to consider a number of possible contributory factors. Clearly, the possibility that the child may have a developmental disorder such as autistic spectrum disorder must be considered. However, some deaf children exhibit restricted play skills or what appears to be an obsessional interest in particular toys, but no other symptoms of developmental delay or ASD. In such cases it is possible that these behaviours are the result of the need or desire for predictability or control in a world in which the child has limited means of exerting control, due to limited communication skills. Alternatively, factors such as cultural practices, social deprivation or parental mental health problems may be influencing the child's early development of play. It is important to bear in mind that not all children have access to rich play opportunities especially if they do not attend any playgroups or other pre-school educational provision and have no siblings, and this can have a significant impact on their opportunities to learn 'how' to play. Cultural factors may be playing an important role here.

Behaviour assessment

Aside from issues around hearing aid compliance, children under the age of two years rarely present with significant behavioural problems. However, from around their second birthday most children become more challenging for their parents to manage behaviourally, as they become more independent and test boundaries. It is important to try to establish whether any behaviours the parents find difficult to manage are simply typical 'toddler' behaviours, or indicative of a more serious, clinical problem, which is likely to impact on progress with a cochlear implant. Parents frequently interpret their child's temper tantrums as resulting from frustration over problems communicating. Whilst this may be true in a proportion of cases, it is much more common for challenging behaviours of this sort to be part of a wider picture of oppositional or non-compliant behaviour. Although it is more difficult to explain to a hearing-impaired child 'why' they should or should not do something, it is rarely impossible to indicate through demonstration, gesture and facial expression 'what' is expected of them. Occasionally, as with hearing aid compliance, difficulty enforcing appropriate boundaries with the child is the result of emotional issues for the parents, relating to the acceptance of their child's deafness, rather than factors intrinsic to the child. For example, some parents express the belief that it is unfair to make their young deaf child do anything he or she doesn't want to do as the child already has enough to cope with being deaf. Such issues require careful and sensitive exploration by the psychologist and suggestions regarding changing the way the parents respond to unwanted behaviours may be met with resistance. However, the importance of such behaviours should not be underestimated in terms of the impact on the child's progress in the long term. Where appropriate, intervention should be offered to the family before their child receives a cochlear implant, in order to minimize any negative impact of behaviour problems.

Aspects of the child's behaviour that should be assessed are summarized below:

- generalized behaviour problems, for example temper tantrums, oppositional behaviour, aggression, toileting, sleep or eating problems

- compliance with adult-directed activities

- difficult behaviours or phobias associated with hospital visits, medical procedures or acceptance of medication

- hearing aid compliance

- attention/hyperactivity problems.

As with any psychological assessment of childhood behaviour problems, behaviour should be considered in all relevant environments – at home, in the educational setting, in the clinic and with other family members and significant caregivers. It can be useful to administer standardized behaviour question-naires as part of the assessment, for example the Child Behaviour Checklist (Achenbach 1991a, 1992), Conners' Rating Scales – Revised (Conners 1997) or the Strengths and Difficulties Questionnaire (Goodman 1997). However, it must be remembered that such questionnaires are not standardized on hearing-impaired children, so any scores derived from them must be interpreted carefully.

Although behaviour problems are very common amongst pre-school-aged deaf children, older deaf children may also present with significant difficulties in this area. Oppositional behaviour, aggression, attention or hyperactivity problems may persist despite the clear boundaries and discipline encountered in the school environment. When such difficulties do persist it often suggests a more significant psychological problem for the child, and may be indicative of underlying cognitive or social communication difficulties. Thorough assess-ment of behaviour problems in this group is essential so that appropriate intervention can be offered and progress with an implant optimized. As with the younger children, observation of the child across settings, a comprehensive history of the problems from parents and other adults who know the child well, along with judicious use of questionnaires, will permit a psychological formulation of the problems to be made.

School-aged children may also occasionally present with symptoms of anxiety or low mood and again a full history should be taken. A number of possible reasons for this type of problem should be explored, including bullying (especially if the child is the only deaf child in his or her class/school), difficul-ties communicating effectively with peers or family, worries about school work, issues around the aetiology of their deafness, their understanding of deafness and their self-concept.

Another area that it is important to explore routinely as part of the pre-implant assessment is the child's previous experiences of hospital visits and medical procedures. Many children have spent much of their early years undergoing investigations and treatments, some of which may have been highly unpleasant or frightening. If this is the case, their ability to cope with cochlear implant assessments, including undergoing general anaesthesia for CT or MRI scans, may be influenced by previous experience. Some children exhibit significant fears or phobias relating to medical procedures, medication or even simply the sight of someone in a white coat or nurse's uniform. If so, the child will need specialist preparation for surgery if he or she is to avoid being traumatized further by cochlear implant surgery.

Additional difficulties assessment

The proportion of hearing-impaired children with disabilities in addition to their deafness has consistently been placed at around 30 to 40 per cent (e.g Fortnum, Marshall and Summerfield 2002; Gallaudet Research Institute 2005). When paediatric cochlear implantation was in its infancy one of the exclusion criteria for the procedure was the presence of additional disabilities. However, in more recent years candidacy criteria have relaxed considerably such that many children with very significant additional disabilities do receive cochlear implants. In these cases the expected outcomes may be in terms of awareness of sounds and improved quality of life rather than aural/oral communication and language skills. It must be remembered that the severity of children's additional difficulties are on a continuum, as are the range of outcomes following cochlear implantation.

Children with complex needs will tend to require a longer assessment for cochlear implantation, as well as different assessment tools and adaptations to their administration, compared with children who are 'only' deaf. For example, a child with a significant visual impairment (deaf-blind) will not be able to undertake a standard test of non-verbal abilities. Yet it is particularly important in such a child to try to establish whether they have the learning ability needed to learn to understand the auditory input provided by a cochlear implant. Whilst evidence suggesting that the child does have the cognitive ability to interpret the auditory stimulus does not guarantee a positive outcome, evidence that the child has significant learning difficulties *is* predictive of a less favourable outcome. In the absence of results from a standardized cognitive assessment the clinical psychologist needs to make a judgement based on observation of the child's play skills – how they explore their environment and novel toys, their ability to learn signs made on their body, and their understanding of cause and effect. Depending on the age of the child it can be useful to set the child and family a learning task during the period of assessment, if it is not possible to gain sufficient evidence during the assessment sessions themselves. For example, the parents (and/or local professionals working with the child) may be asked to teach the child to sort objects by shape or size, or semantic category (e.g. fruits). It may be possible to administer some sections of an appropriate developmental assessment. In visually impaired children one such instrument is the Reynell-Zinkin Scales for Young Visually Handicapped Children (Reynell 1979), from which the Social Adaptation, Sensorimotor Understanding and Exploration of Environment sections can be used and provide useful information.

In children with a dual sensory loss, or other additional disabilities, factors other than the child's cognitive abilities may influence the potential benefit to be achieved following cochlear implantation. Many deaf-blind children exhibit challenging behaviours, including obsessional behaviours and self-harm. These can make engaging the child in the necessary (re)habilitation activities very difficult, or even impossible. This must be taken into consideration when deciding whether a cochlear implant is an appropriate intervention.

Other types of complex needs will also require an individually tailored assessment protocol. Children with cerebral palsy or other motor/physical disabilities may be able to attempt a test such as the Leiter-R, but are likely to need the psychologist (and indeed other members of the team when assessing the child) to explore alternative response modes, for example pointing to the correct response card rather than moving it into place, or by using eye-pointing. Creativity on the part of the psychologist is essential when working with these children.

A further potential presentation of a child with additional difficulties is one whose communication skills are atypical even taking into account their hearing loss. Concerns about autistic spectrum behaviours will need to be followed up appropriately either by referral to a specialist ASD service local to where the child lives, or to one based within the same hospital as the Cochlear Implant Programme, where this is available. Occasionally it may also be the case that members of the Cochlear Implant Programme team are suitably trained and experienced to make the diagnosis. Autism and deafness are explored fully in Chapter 5, and we would refer the reader there for further information on this topic. The issues relating to assessment of children with complex needs for cochlear implantation, along with a review of the literature regarding outcomes following the procedure are provided by Edwards (2007).

Assessment of self-concept and self-esteem

On the whole, congenitally profoundly deaf children are not considered suitable candidates for cochlear implantation after the age of six to seven years, as the hearing nerve has not been adequately stimulated and therefore loses the capacity to transmit meaningful signals to the brain. Children in this category are almost never able to discuss how they see themselves or feel about themselves as they have neither the cognitive maturity nor language skills to do so. However, it is appropriate for older children who have either had a progressive hearing loss or lost their hearing through illness or injury, to present for cochlear implant assessment. In these cases it is very important to allow the child or adolescent to reflect on their experience of being deaf and how they feel about themselves and their deafness.

As children progress through their teenage years they increasingly compare themselves with others. Deaf children considering cochlear implantation may compare themselves with hearing or deaf peers, the latter either with or without hearing aids or cochlear implants. Not surprisingly these comparisons are based on the child's knowledge of other individuals, particularly children at school. Given that there is a wide variety of cognitive and communication abilities amongst children with hearing aids or cochlear implants, some cochlear implant candidates may have negative perceptions of cochlear implant users. In these circumstances it is helpful to introduce the cochlear implant candidate to an implant recipient who has as much in common with them as possible, in terms of age, cause of deafness, general ability and so on.

It is important to be mindful that for some families seeking a cochlear implant, issues around a culturally Deaf identity may be relevant, and need to be explored sensitively.

Some children and adolescents express concern that a cochlear implant may fundamentally 'change' them, or their personality, in some way. They may question whether the proximity of the internal parts of the implant to the brain means that the brain or mind will be negatively affected by the procedure. Thankfully it is possible to fully reassure them that no harmful effects of this sort have ever been documented, or even reported anecdotally.

Decision to implant and consent

After all the relevant assessments and investigations have been completed it is usual for all the members of the Cochlear Implant Programme team involved to meet to discuss their findings and consider whether a cochlear implant is an appropriate intervention for that particular child. The crux of the issue is whether a cochlear implant is likely to provide the child with better auditory information than the most appropriate hearing aids, taking into consideration factors intrinsic to the child and factors relating to the child's family, social and educational circumstances. Most Paediatric Cochlear Implant Programme teams use a version of the Children's Implant Profile (ChIP), originally devised by Hellman *et al.* (1991), to guide their decision-making. The profile comprises a number of factors, typically between 12 and 18, each of which is rated on a three-point scale: 'no concern', 'mild–moderate concern', and 'great concern', in terms of the impact on potential benefit from the implant. Definitions or criteria for what constitutes each level of concern have evolved over the past 15 years or so, as research has sought to identify predictors of benefit. As a result, each team is likely to use slightly different criteria. No score is derived from the profile and therefore there is no 'cut-off' beyond which a child is considered unsuitable. Some factors are more predictive of speech outcomes than others and therefore these would need to be weighted to reflect this. However, at present there is little scientific evidence to determine such a weighting system and although each rating is based on specific criteria, judgements for many of them are subjective. Therefore, it would not be ethical to base a decision purely on a numerical figure. Also, some considerations may override all others, as for example in the case of children with Usher syndrome who will lose their sight, and therefore be reliant on whatever auditory input they can receive.

Where concerns are raised by the team it is often possible to work with the child and family to improve the likelihood of a positive outcome with an implant. Factors that are likely to be included in some format on the ChIP are:

- age

- radiological and anatomical findings

- medical consideration

- audiological findings

- use of hearing aids

- communication skills (signed and/or oral)

- cognitive ability/general development

- behaviour

- family structure and support

- expectations

- educational environment and availability of support services (speech and language therapy and teachers of the deaf)

- learning style

- attendance/ease of access to cochlear implant centre.

Recent research has shown that one of the strongest predictors of progress with a cochlear implant is global developmental delay or general cognitive ability (e.g. Edwards, Frost and Witham 2006). Therefore, information from the psychological assessment is an essential part of the decision-making process. Where the decision is that a cochlear implant is likely to be of benefit to the child, this is usually greeted with pleasure and relief by the child's family. Most parents accept the earliest possible date for surgery and eagerly await the 'switch-on' sessions. However, for some parents the decision is not straightforward even if the Cochlear Implant Programme team considers a cochlear implant to be in the child's best interests. There are many possible reasons for parents' reservations, including fears about the long anaesthetic required for surgery, potential surgical risks and complications, other medical problems, family and cultural attitudes and implications for schooling. Given that the procedure is an elective one, for a non-life-threatening condition, parents do, of course, have the right to choose not to follow the team's recommendation. In this context it is important to ensure that both parents are in agreement with the decision. Legal issues are also relevant, as consent for the operation must be sought from an adult with 'parental responsibility' for the child, and where differences in opinion exist this has the potential to lead to court proceedings. In practice, in our experience the situation has been resolved before reaching such an extreme scenario. Counselling by the psychologist may be necessary to help families arrive at a final decision about whether a cochlear implant is what they want for their child.

Although the vast majority of children who are assessed for cochlear implantation do go on to receive one, there are circumstances where the cochlear implant team feel that an implant is not in the child's best interests. Severe learning difficulties, some medical conditions and other complex needs may mean that the risks of the procedure and the long-term commitment to appointments and rehabilitation required outweigh the potential benefits. This is often very hard for parents to accept as they may perceive the implant as being the solution to many, if not all, their child's difficulties. Again, it may be necessary for the psychologist to offer support to parents at this time, and explore alternative options, including referral to other services such as specialist communication clinics or diagnostic services.

In young deaf children the issue of consent to surgery is rarely complex, as the parent(s) of the child will automatically make the decision on behalf of the child and sign the consent forms for surgery. Although members of the Deaf community have argued that parents should wait until their child is able to decide whether they want an implant and consent to the surgery for themselves, this is not viable. If we were to wait for a (congenitally) deaf child to have developed the level of cognitive functioning required to give truly informed consent, the benefit to be gained from a cochlear implant in terms of oral/aural language development would almost certainly be negligible. Thus, in the pre-school child, parents (or those with parental responsibility) provide consent and the child may have little or no understanding of the implications of the decision for the immediate or long-term future.

In contrast, in older children and adolescents, the issue of consent to surgery, and indeed the entire process from assessment to long-term follow-up, becomes very pertinent. It is not unusual for the child to have significant reservations about the surgery in particular and they may need considerable reassurance about its safety, levels of pain to be expected and so on. Children should be given as much information as they want about the hospital stay and operation, at a level appropriate to their age, language and cognitive abilities. Visual aids to understanding are an important part of this, as is a visit to the ward where they will be looked after. If the team is satisfied that the child is fully informed about the likely benefit for them of having an implant, is equally informed regarding the consequences of *not* having an implant, and the child does not consent to the procedure, it is not appropriate for the operation to go ahead.

Case example: Consent to treatment and preparation

A ten-year-old boy, Samir, with a progressive hearing loss associated with widened vestibular aqueduct syndrome presented for assessment for cochlear implantation. His parents reported that over the previous six months his school work had deteriorated, his speech intelligibility had worsened noticeably and he was becoming increasingly withdrawn and uncharacteristically 'moody'. He attended a mainstream school with limited support from specialist teachers of the deaf, and was becoming isolated from his peers, particularly in social situations. On completion of the ChIP, the main areas of concern noted were the lack of appropriate educational support for his changing needs and the expectations of both Samir and his parents – Samir stated that he didn't believe a cochlear implant would make any difference to his ability to hear, whilst his parents felt that an implant would make him hear 'normally', equally well as his hearing peers.

The implant team considered Samir to be a very good candidate for cochlear implantation and explained to him the improvements in detecting speech sounds he could expect using an implant, based on his current audiogram. However, Samir was very adamant that he did not want an implant as he felt that he was coping well with his hearing aids. This surprised and perplexed his parents (and the implant team). Samir was offered a number of appointments with the team's clinical psychologist to further explore his understanding of what a cochlear implant can/cannot and does/does not do, and his feelings about becoming profoundly deaf after many years of coping with some hearing. Initially Samir was reluctant to attend the sessions, until he was reassured that their purpose was not to persuade him, or worse still 'force' him to have an implant, as he believed. It emerged that he had a significant phobia of blood that he had not mentioned to anyone, feared being teased, and also was highly anxious about being anaesthetized as a result of a previous negative experience. Following a number of further sessions to address these areas of concern using a cognitive-behavioural framework, Samir consented to the surgery, which proceeded uneventfully.

Switch-on and post-implant

The main part of this chapter has focused on the assessment of whether a cochlear implant is an appropriate intervention for a child, specifically from psychological and social perspectives. However, there are a number of further areas of involvement for psychologists, once the child has undergone the implant surgery.

The process of 'switch-on', when the implant is activated for the first time, is primarily the responsibility of the audiologists on the implant team, but is also often done jointly with speech and language therapists or teachers of the deaf who will start the long process of helping the child to develop 'listening skills'. Switch-on typically involves more than one session and very occasionally a child may react negatively to their first experience of sound. If the response is so severe that rejection of the device is a possibility, the psychologist's input may be sought, for example to advise on a graded programme of increasing tolerance of the implant. Sometimes this means starting from the point where the child is willing to look at the speech processor and coil in their box although thankfully this degree of fear of the implant is very rare.

Sometimes children appear to have accepted the implant well initially, only to stop using it after a number of weeks, months or even years. The reasons underlying rejection of the implant may be relatively simple, for example as a way of ensuring parental attention by a toddler, or highly complex, as in the case of an adolescent who is being bullied at school and is questioning his or her identity as a deaf individual. The role of the psychologist may involve working with the child's parents in implementing a behavioural programme for a young child where non-use of the implant is part of a picture of general non-compliance. Equally, the psychologist may need to work psychotherapeutically with an adolescent who has poor self-esteem and difficulties with peer relationships. Although issues around identity and self-concept may be associated with reluctance to use the implant, older children and adolescents may need the opportunity to explore these areas even if they are happy with their cochlear implant. They may have questions about the cause of their deafness, why they have an implant (as opposed to conventional hearing aids), whether they will ever be able to hear 'normally' or even whether, if they have children, they too will be deaf.

There are two other primary reasons why psychological input may be required for a child with a cochlear implant – emotional and/or behavioural problems or specific learning difficulties resulting in lack of progress in developing listening, communication, language, literacy or numeracy skills to the expected level. These topics are covered in separate chapters and therefore will not be considered further here, except to say that the process of assessing a specific learning difficulty in a child with a cochlear implant is essentially the same as that for a hearing-impaired child with hearing aids. Referral for these problems may be made at any point after the child has received the cochlear implant, even many years later, and may be made by other members of the Cochlear Implant Programme team, local professionals or the parents of the child.

Finally, it is good practice for implant team psychologists to offer review appointments, usually around the first anniversary of switch-on, and possibly at specified intervals thereafter. Times of transition, for example from primary to secondary education, or from the Paediatric Cochlear Implant Programme to an adult one, are likely to be points at which the child and his or her family may value the opportunity to reflect on progress with the implant, any psychological or learning problems, and hopes and aspirations for the future. It may be necessary to ensure the young adult has access to appropriate psychological services once they have moved on from the Paediatric Cochlear Implant Programme. Where issues around transition occur, for example meeting special educational needs arising from additional difficulties, changes in peer group or high levels of child anxiety or distress, close liaison between the implant team psychologist and local educational, social and psychological services may be required.

Conclusions

The involvement of psychologists in the field of cochlear implantation is still comparatively rare, particularly in the UK. However, we hope that this chapter has given a flavour of the input that psychologists can offer implant teams and the children and families who access their services. The world of cochlear implantation is a fast-changing one, and we have no desire to be prescriptive about the roles and activities of psychologists in this context, as these will undoubtedly change over time. Indeed, in this chapter we have only discussed the clinical work a psychologist may be requested to offer; research, teaching and training of psychologists and other professionals, and consultancy all form exciting, challenging aspects of the work of psychologists in cochlear implantation, but have not been included here.

7 Tinnitus

Tinnitus in children is a much more common problem than generally realized and is especially prevalent amongst hearing-impaired children and adolescents. Unfortunately, it frequently goes unrecognized in children (and therefore untreated). In this chapter we will begin with a description of what constitutes tinnitus, its clinical presentation and what is known about its causes. Consideration of the epidemiology of tinnitus in children, how it is diagnosed and the impact it has on children's lives will follow. Traditional interventions will also be briefly outlined. One of the psychological approaches that has received attention in adult tinnitus sufferers and been found to be effective is cognitive-behavioural therapy (CBT). Many of the strategies incorporated in this approach can be adapted for older children and adolescents, for example education about tinnitus, relaxation and challenging negative beliefs about tinnitus. Cognitive-behavioural therapy in younger deaf children (and to some extent all young children) can be problematical due to the limited language skills of many of them. Therefore, the main focus of the chapter will be on an alternative therapeutic approach that we have found valuable in working with hearing children and those with a permanent hearing-impairment who are experiencing disabling tinnitus – narrative therapy. We will briefly outline some of the central tenets of the approach along with how these can be applied to children with tinnitus, through a number of clinical case examples.

Clinical presentation and aetiology

The term tinnitus refers to the sensation or perception of hearing a noise when there is no external sound present. It may be experienced as being in one or both ears or in the middle of the head. Some individuals find it difficult to give an exact location. The noises are described in a wide variety of ways – as high, medium or low pitched, as a buzzing, ringing or humming sound, loud or quiet or as a single sound or a sound with different components. Tinnitus may be experienced as constantly present, intermittent and fluctuating in duration and intensity.

It is important to remember that tinnitus is not a disease or illness, rather it is a symptom that is generated within the auditory neural pathways. Tinnitus may occasionally arise as a result of disease of the ears, and is associated with sensori-neural hearing loss. A number of treatment-induced (iatrogenic) causes have been noted, for example drug-induced ototoxicity resulting from the use of drugs such as aspirin, quinine and some chemotherapeutic agents. However, it is much more commonly associated with exposure to loud noise, especially music, in young people. Tinnitus may also be triggered by a head injury, meningitis or surgery to the inner ear (Aust 2002). Holgers and Juul (2006) note that predisposing factors for greater severity of tinnitus are high-frequency hearing loss and anxiety and depressive disorders. However, in a great many cases of childhood tinnitus, no cause can be identified.

In terms of the mechanism by which tinnitus is generated, there are a number of theories. For example, Jastreboff (1990) proposed a 'neurophysiological model of tinnitus' where the tinnitus results from abnormal processing of a signal generated in the auditory system. Such models emphasize the relationship between activity in the prefrontal cortex and limbic systems of the brain. Since the limbic system mediates emotions, this may help account for the high levels of distress experienced by many tinnitus sufferers, and the high levels of anxiety and depression in this group of patients. However, this is less helpful in understanding tinnitus in hearing-impaired children, who tend not to complain spontaneously of the symptom and are less likely to be distressed by it.

Given that tinnitus is such a subjective experience it is difficult to gain accurate information regarding its severity in individual cases. Reporting of symptoms generally by children is notoriously unreliable, especially in young children, and this makes assessing tinnitus in children a challenge. However, at a clinical level, the severity of symptoms in a particular child relative to that of other children, or in comparison with the maximum possible severity is irrelevant: it is the extent to which the child is affected by his or her symptoms and his or her life is disrupted that matters.

Epidemiology

Studies examining the incidence or prevalence of tinnitus in children are few and mostly relatively recent. Reported rates of tinnitus in children with sensori-neural hearing loss (SNHL) vary widely overall from around one-quarter to two-thirds of children, depending on the criteria used for diagnosing tinnitus, the age of the children and the degree of consistency of response required of the child. However, there are indications that the prevalence of tinnitus is greater in children with a moderate–severe hearing impairment than those with a profound loss (e.g. Graham and Butler 1984; Nodar and Lezak 1984). Research suggests that children with SNHL rarely complain of tinnitus spontaneously (e.g. Mills, Albert and Brain 1986; Nodar and Lezak 1984; Savastano 2007). In a large-scale study of 1420 children with either a suspicion or previous history of hearing disorder, Aust (2002) found that 7 per cent of the children had experienced tinnitus, and nearly three-quarters of these had objective hearing loss. Studies on the prevalence of tinnitus in children with SNHL compared with children with normal hearing produce conflicting results. For example, Stouffer *et al.* (1992) found a lower prevalence in children with normal hearing of between 6 and 13 per cent, compared with 24–29 per cent in those with a hearing-impairment. Other studies have found remarkably similar rates between the two groups, for example Mills and Cherry (1984) provide figures of 29 per cent and 29.5 per cent for normally hearing and hearing-impaired children respectively, and Holgers (2003) reported 13 per cent and 9 per cent respectively. Savastano (2007) also found no relationship between the presence of tinnitus and severity of hearing loss.

A number of authors have suggested that children with tinnitus rarely complain about it and that they are more tolerant of a regular aural sensation than the adult population. It has also been suggested that children may not realize that other people do not hear sounds in this way and therefore do not perceive them as abnormal. The number of children spontaneously complaining of tinnitus has been placed at only around 3 per cent by Mills *et al.* (1986) and 6.5 per cent by Savastano (2007), but when children do mention it of their own accord, it is likely that the tinnitus is causing distress and should therefore be taken seriously.

Impact of tinnitus in children

Very few researchers have attempted to identify which factors predict the severity of tinnitus. In adults there appears to be a stronger relationship between the severity of symptoms and psychological factors such as anxiety, depression, concentration problems and irritability, than between symptoms and audiological status (see Holgers, Erlandsson and Barrenas 2000 for a review). Early studies tended to focus on how 'troublesome' or 'annoying' the tinnitus was. Tyler and Baker (1983) surveyed 72 adults with tinnitus and found that the condition was associated with hearing difficulties in 53 per cent, lifestyle was affected in 93 per cent, general health in 56 per cent and emotional difficulties were reported in 70 per cent of the sample. Getting to sleep was the most frequently mentioned difficulty and many respondents indicated that they experienced depression, annoyance and insecurity. Complaints relating to sleep disturbance, auditory interference and emotional distress have been consistently found in subsequent studies (Hallam 1987; Sanchez and Stephens 1997). These now seem to be clearly established domains of complaint for adult tinnitus sufferers.

Little is known, however, about the ways in which tinnitus is troublesome for children, and the impact it has upon their lives. Graham (1987) acknowledges that the degree of annoyance caused by tinnitus in hearing-impaired children can be difficult to assess, but found that in one-third of hearing-impaired children in their study the tinnitus could be described as annoying. Aksoy *et al.* (2007) assessed 1039 school-aged children and reported that 39 per cent of the 157 children with tinnitus described it as disturbing and 38 per cent of them said it interfered with their sleep and caused difficulty concentrating. A small number of children report being severely worried by the symptom (5%), but 42 per cent are worried by it to some extent (Savastano 2007). Martin and Snashall (1994) completed a retrospective multi-centre survey of 42 children who had attended an audiology clinic complaining of tinnitus. Approximately 50 per cent of their sample of children with tinnitus had normal hearing, and in those with a hearing impairment, all degrees of hearing loss were represented. Overall, they found that 83 per cent of the children reported their tinnitus as troublesome and a close relationship between tinnitus and other associated symptoms, that is, dizziness and headaches was reported. Twelve of the children complained that tinnitus interfered with their sleep, six highlighted difficulties in concentrating, and five children reported stress or fatigue. They concluded that there is a sub-population of children who experience tinnitus for whom the problem is just as severe as it can be in adults.

Drukier (1989) reported that 70 per cent of children with a severe to profound hearing loss had difficulties understanding speech when their tinnitus was present. This has been suggested to contribute to behavioural problems, including poor attentiveness and poor school performance.

Kentish, Crocker and McKenna (2000) described a small-scale study that looked at 24 children (12 with normal hearing and 12 with a hearing loss) who presented to the psychology department of a specialist audiology centre with troublesome tinnitus. Results suggest that tinnitus can have as marked an impact on children's lives as it is reported to have on adults. Insomnia, emotional distress, listening and attention difficulties were found to be the main psychological factors associated with tinnitus in children. These in turn may have an effect upon their school performance. Differences were found between children with normal hearing and those with some degree of hearing loss. Overall, children with normal hearing seemed to find tinnitus more troublesome than those with some level of hearing-impairment, and thus tinnitus appears to have a bigger psychological impact on hearing children. The study suggested that children who complain of tinnitus should be taken seriously as the potential sequaelae are considerable.

More recently, Holgers and Juul (2006) assessed tinnitus severity in 95 children and young people aged 8–20 years who were attending a tinnitus clinic in Sweden. They used a questionnaire that comprised items addressing the impact of tinnitus on concentration, sleep, mood, quality of life and the ability to 'mask' tinnitus. They also used visual analogue scales to measure the loudness (ranging from no perception of sound to extremely strong perception of sound) and annoyance/degree of disturbance (ranging from didn't disturb at all to unbearable) of the tinnitus. Finally, they asked their participants to complete the Hospital Anxiety and Depression Scale (HAD; Zigmond and Snaith 1983), an adult measure that has been validated for use with children and adolescents (White et al. 1999). Holgers and Juul report a weak but significant correlation between degree of high-frequency hearing loss and severity of tinnitus, and stronger correlations between degree of high-frequency hearing loss and the loudness and annoyance of the tinnitus. Severity of tinnitus was related to the severity of anxiety and depression. Of importance was the finding that amongst adolescents, approximately one-third scored above the cut-off level for possible or probable clinical anxiety and 15 per cent for clinical depression. Of course, causality cannot be inferred from this finding, and indeed it could be argued that the relationship between tinnitus and disorders of mood occurs in either direction, or both.

Results from the Kentish et al. study (2000) suggest that tinnitus can be a cause of great distress and worry both for children and their families. In line with Tyler and Baker's study (1983), the biggest impact upon children's lives was found to be sleep disturbance, with over three-quarters of the children reporting this as their main concern. It is also interesting to note that only 25 per cent of children were reported as having behavioural problems, although almost two-thirds of the sample of normally hearing children showed clear symptoms of anxiety. Although this group of children appear to show signs of distress more through internalizing their feelings rather than through externalizing behaviours, more research is needed to clarify this relationship.

For almost half of the normally hearing children, additional complaints included difficulties listening both at home and at school, difficulties with background noise and attention and concentration difficulties in school. Children with a hearing loss reported fewer difficulties in these domains, which was an unexpected finding. One possible explanation may be that children with some degree of hearing-impairment may be more accustomed to auditory distur- bance and thus find the impact of tinnitus less disruptive. This is a tentative finding on a small sample of children, and future research will hopefully help to shed further light on this observation.

Finally, in this study, just over half the sample of children reported specific worries about tinnitus, for example that it might be damaging, or reflecting deterioration in their hearing. These fears were equally shared by the parents. In some cases, children had personified their tinnitus noises into frightening char- acters. It was difficult to estimate the onset point, or the frequency of tinnitus in most children, as the younger children were unable to give reliable estimates of time.

Traditional interventions

When tinnitus is considered troublesome by the child, advice from the medical profession may be sought. Although there is rarely a medical or physical cause for the tinnitus that can be 'cured', it is always advisable for the child to be assessed by a specialist ENT doctor. If a specific problem with the ear(s) is iden- tified, this can be treated appropriately. It is also usual for the child's hearing to be checked and if a significant hearing loss is found, hearing aids may be fitted. Correcting the hearing loss may have an indirect, positive impact on the tinnitus since, by allowing the child to hear everyday sounds (including speech) more easily, these sounds may become more distinguishable from the tinnitus, thereby reducing perception of the tinnitus. Thus, where needed, hearing aids may help the brain to filter out the unwanted sounds and make it easier to focus on external sounds.

Once the possibility of a treatable cause has been eliminated, intervention typically focuses initially on information, explanation and reassurance. Children may have fears that there is a sinister cause for their symptoms. Reassurance that this is not the case, along with explaining what is known about tinnitus, may reduce any distress associated with the symptom. In particular, knowing that help is available and that the symptom is unlikely to be permanent generates a sense of hope that is therapeutic in its own right.

The use of tinnitus 'maskers', or white noise generators may help some young people with tinnitus. These small electronic devices produce a quiet external sound that allows the child to concentrate less on the internal tinnitus sounds. Other sounds, if used regularly, can produce a similar effect (i.e. habitua- tion to the tinnitus sounds), for example quiet background music, a fan or other quiet sound of the child's choice. Tinnitus is often more noticeable or troublesome when in a quiet situation, the most obvious of which is when trying to go to sleep. Careful use of sounds at this time may be beneficial.

Finally, children may find it helpful to learn relaxation techniques, especially if they identify that their tinnitus is exacerbated by stress. Keeping a diary of stress levels, tiredness or other possible influencing factors, and the severity of their tinnitus, may highlight triggers or exacerbating factors, which can be improved by relaxation and stress-relieving techniques.

These strategies are ones 'borrowed' from those typically used with adult tinnitus sufferers. In recent years, these broadly psychological strategies have been added to in the form of a more systematic, theory-driven psychological approach, that of cognitive-behavioural therapy (CBT). CBT for adult tinnitus patients involves a combination of strategies, typically including education (about tinnitus and the link between thoughts and feelings arising from the experience of tinnitus), challenging unhelpful beliefs and assumptions about tinnitus, and behavioural testing of hypotheses regarding these beliefs. Relaxation and imagery techniques along with exposure to exacerbating situations whilst employing learnt coping strategies to promote habituation are also used.

A small number of empirical studies have examined the effectiveness of CBT for adult tinnitus sufferers. In a Cochrane Review of available randomized, controlled trials of CBT, Martinez Devesa *et al.* (2007) identified six studies, and concluded that, although CBT did not have an impact on the patients' subjective tinnitus loudness or level of depression, it did have a significant positive impact on quality of life (a decrease in global tinnitus severity).

There is no equivalent research base in children. In the following sections, we will present an alternative therapeutic approach that we have found effective in helping young children with tinnitus who are distressed by their symptoms or whose symptoms are having a significant negative impact on their lives: narrative therapy. Although this therapeutic approach will be seen to bear a number of similarities to CBT for tinnitus, it also employs distinct methodologies of its own.

Background to narrative therapy

Stories are an integral part of young children's lives. In narrative therapy we work with the stories children and families tell us about tinnitus along with their thoughts and feelings about it. We look at how tinnitus impacts upon their lives, and how life impacts upon their tinnitus. Often their story is alive with negative connotations and emotions – tinnitus can be frightening. By changing a child's story about tinnitus, we help them to see it in a new light.

The child's family will also have a story about tinnitus as they try to make sense of the child's experience, and how it has impacted upon their lives. Although this story may or may not be the same as the child's, it will be equally alive. When the dominant story lies with the parents, this becomes the focus of intervention. Stories about tinnitus are also connected to the wider system around the child. Significant or upsetting events in a child's life, either at home or at school, can become attached to their story about tinnitus. Tinnitus may be seen as the cause of these difficulties, or as a consequence.

Psychological work with children cannot be too prescriptive. Intervention must be tailored to the child's developmental level and follow a thorough assessment. Intervention packages also need to be tailored to the individual child, and take account of their age, audiological status and life circumstances. Intervention may include individual therapy with the child, work with the family, or school. We use a wide range of intervention strategies, including relaxation techniques and educational assessment. In this chapter however, we focus upon therapeutic techniques for working with the pre-adolescent child. Whilst there are well-developed techniques for working with adults, little attention has been paid to developing techniques for children. Inevitably, this is a more complex area. Young children do not have all the cognitive sophistication required for cognitive-behavioural therapy. The ability to reflect upon their cognitions and emotions does not develop until late childhood. Nevertheless, we assume many of the same principles: tinnitus is affected by thoughts and feelings.

What is narrative therapy?

Stories are our most familiar means of communicating the meaning we find in our experiences. Each of us holds stories about ourselves that help us to make sense of our life experiences, and these in turn have the effect of filtering an individual's experience, and thereby selecting what information gets focused in or filtered out (Sween 1999). The narratives we hold about ourselves help us to make sense of what happens to us. For each of us, our lives will be defined by how we respond to the experiences in our lives, as much as by the experiences themselves.

By looking at the stories and meanings associated with tinnitus, narrative therapy helps start to disentangle why it is that for some children and families, tinnitus becomes problematic, and for others it is a matter of little or no consequence. Stories about tinnitus held by children and families will be in part construed from their own personal experiences, but will also be gained from the wider system within which they live. These influences include:

- *Society*: Within the child's society there are commonly held beliefs about tinnitus that the child and family may have heard from health, media, deafness or hearing groups. These beliefs can have a powerful

influence upon how the family approach tinnitus. Such beliefs may
be that tinnitus is only associated with hearing loss; that it does not
occur in children; that tinnitus is a permanent or untreatable
condition.

- *Community, school and friends*: If we look at the influence of
  community, school and friends, we can see that meanings and beliefs
  from these will be important in shaping the family's ideas about
  childhood tinnitus. A teacher for example, who has personal
  experience of tinnitus, will respond to a child's tinnitus quite
  differently from one who knows little about it. A hearing-impaired
  child may be more likely than a hearing one to come into contact
  with another child who has tinnitus, and may be exposed to beliefs
  about tinnitus that are inaccurate or unhelpful.

- *The family*: Family stories about illness, hearing-impairment, and
  hospitals will have a bearing on how treatment is approached. For
  example, whether the child feels believed or understood by their
  family, and feels that the tinnitus is taken seriously, will affect their
  response to it and their coping strategies. Conversely, if the child's
  family believe tinnitus is an illness or results from a sinister cause, the
  child will develop a different set of emotional and behavioural
  responses.

- *The child*: Children are influenced by the meanings and beliefs
  conveyed by the wider system around them, and even very young
  children will pick up their parents' responses to illness, hospitals and
  tinnitus. The exact nature and interpretation of these meanings and
  beliefs will depend on the developmental level of the child, their
  cognitive abilities and language skills. A commonly held view is that
  talking to a child about his or her tinnitus may make it worse. A
  tinnitus consultation may therefore be the first time that a child has
  been allowed to voice his or her concerns in a developmentally
  appropriate way.

Interviewing the young child

With young children, it is important not to apply the 'child as a small adult' way
of thinking. Developmental change is extensive within childhood. The child's
level of language, cognitive and social development will impact upon their
understanding of tinnitus, their ability to describe it, and to participate in different kinds of treatment. Research on children's pain suggests that by around

seven years of age, children can give reasonably sophisticated descriptions of their pain, although it remains impossible to know whether a 'nagging' pain for one child feels the same as a nagging pain for another child. The experience of tinnitus is likely to be equally difficult for young children to describe and quantify, particularly for hearing-impaired children whose language skills may be significantly delayed compared with their hearing peers. Adult-like (abstract and complex) understanding of illness does not occur until adolescence. The child's cognitive and developmental status will therefore influence the level of sophistication of illness concepts and pain-related beliefs, and by analogy, tinnitus-related beliefs. Children may generate their own hypotheses and explanations for the causes of their pain, illness or symptoms, in the absence of information that is complete, or has been given at a developmentally inappropriate level. Children will thus construct their own 'stories' to account for their tinnitus.

To understand the child's story about tinnitus, we need as much information as possible about their tinnitus. Play and drawing are useful ways for young children to depict their ideas and feelings about tinnitus, particularly when language skills are limited. Most children enjoy drawing. A picture of what tinnitus looks like can be highly revealing, and a useful starting point to the process of externalization (this concept is explained in a later section).

Medical professionals often adopt a closed form of questioning, requiring a yes/no form of answer that is likely to limit the information the child spontaneously provides. Indeed, it has been shown that young children will often answer a nonsense question when presented in a closed format (e.g. 'Which is pink: a tree or a bee?'). Children will often try to please adults by providing the answer they think the adult wants to hear. In contrast, we know that children generate more information from open-ended questions. A young child may not be able to describe his or her tinnitus in a temporal way. Frequency and duration are hard for the young child to assess or recall. This information does need to be gathered, and it is best done through a recording chart over a period of time. Younger children are less able to link tinnitus to events, feelings or internal cognitions (e.g. what thoughts are triggered when the tinnitus is intrusive) or their mood. As part of ongoing therapy, these connections need to be taught through intervention, or through observations of their behaviour when tinnitus occurs.

The initial interview

At the initial interview, all the family is invited to the appointment. The child and therapist can complete further information booklets (see Kentish and Crocker 2005) that serve the function of gathering information about the child's understanding of his or her tinnitus and hearing, and factors that influence it. Past and present strategies for managing the child's tinnitus are explored. This is an important part of the assessment as many families come to the first appointment believing that they have tried all the possible interventions for tinnitus, and that they have been referred for psychological input because the medical professionals think their child is at best exaggerating the problem, or at worst 'mad'. Identification of strategies that have alleviated the tinnitus begins the process of changing the dominant story about tinnitus; the child and parent can begin to see that tinnitus is not something to be passively endured.

Formal measures (questionnaires) of anxiety and depression can also be used. If necessary, the therapist will go through these with the child, depending upon their age.

The remainder of the interview is used to map the influence of tinnitus upon the child, and vice versa. Other events in the child's life are explored with the child, their parents and siblings as appropriate. We are interested to know why the child's tinnitus has become troublesome at this point in time, precipitating a referral, and whether there are particular events either at home or school that may be affecting the child. Common events include: school examinations, difficulty getting on with the teacher, difficulties with academic work; and at home, marital or other family difficulties, health problems in another family member, or bereavement.

Assessment and formulation
Information gathering
Information is gathered about the child's tinnitus through multiple methods. Before the first appointment, the school can be contacted for information about the child's educational progress, friendships or any other difficulties noted by the child's teacher. Parents can be sent a questionnaire (see Kentish and Crocker 2005), which begins to focus in upon their understanding of the child's tinnitus, and factors contributing to it. By the end of the initial assessment it should be possible to answer the following questions:

- Can the child's tinnitus be described (e.g. frequency, times of the day when it is most likely to occur, what it sounds like, any triggers)?

- Are there other associated health and psychological problems (headaches, dizziness, hyperacusis [heightened sensitivity to sound])?

- How does the tinnitus influence the child's daily life (sleep difficulties, anxiety, depression, irritability)?

- Does the tinnitus influence the child's school life (e.g. difficulties listening or concentrating in class)?

- How does the tinnitus influence friendships and family?

- Are there current life events that have influenced tinnitus (e.g. family or school difficulties)?

- What do the child, family and teacher know about tinnitus? How correct is this information?

- What are the beliefs within the family about the child's tinnitus (e.g. the child is going deaf; child has a brain tumour)?

- Who in the family is most worried about the child's tinnitus (parent or child)?

- What stories does the family have about illness, hospitals and hearing loss?

- Can situations or thoughts that contradict the dominant tinnitus story be identified?

- Coping strategies: what has the child tried to do already to alleviate the tinnitus? Has this been successful?

- What have the parents tried to do to help their child? What effect has this had?

Intervention and narrative therapy techniques

Next, we begin to unpick the tinnitus story. For each child and family, the dominant story may lie in one or a number of the areas described above. Through assessment, we will have determined where intervention needs to be focused.

Fears and worries about tinnitus

Providing the child and parents with factual information about tinnitus is often the first major turning point. This begins to answer worries such as: 'Is my child going deaf?' Negative beliefs and feelings of hopelessness are commonly part of the story, for example 'I will always have tinnitus and there is nothing I can do about it.' This may have been engendered by parts of the child's system including medical professionals, as in the example of David below.

> **Case example: A story of fear**
>
> Nine-year-old David had a mild to moderate hearing loss. Due to an ear infection he was prescribed a course of antibiotics from his medical practitioner. Whilst the ear infection cleared up, David developed a buzzing in both of his ears. Shortly after, tinnitus was diagnosed by his ENT surgeon. He and his mother were told that there was nothing that could be done about it, and he must 'go away and learn to live with it'. David and his mother were devastated by this. Over the forthcoming weeks he became increasingly distressed, stopped sleeping and attending school.
>
> Information about tinnitus began to focus upon changing the story for David and his mother. First, they were reassured that there was much that could be done to help with the tinnitus. Changing this aspect of the story had a powerful effect for David, and gave a story of hope.

Life stressors linked to tinnitus

If there is an obvious association between an external life event and onset of troublesome tinnitus, then this will clearly need to be addressed, as will any educational or family difficulties.

Individual therapy with the child

Through discussion and play, the aim is to find out what the child's tinnitus sounds like to the child, how it makes them feel and any images it conjures for them. Second, powerful characters or images are sought and explored that will help the child to see tinnitus in a different way, and give them a sense of being in control. During the interview with the child, their response to various activities are closely observed to see which works best for them.

The word tinnitus may be new to the child, and so first it is important to find out whether the child already has his or her own name for it. If not, they can be asked what they would like to call it, and this should be stuck to. The child is asked to draw a picture of tinnitus. For those keen on drawing, this will be both pleasurable and engaging, and often also works well with the older child. The child is invited to play with a collection of toys. Depending upon the age of the child, these will include soft toys, miniature people, Lego and the latest cartoon and Disney characters. It is helpful to have a collection of less friendly looking toys (a 'monster' collection). The child is asked about activities that they enjoy doing at home, whether they have a favourite cartoon, or superhero. Strong, powerful images for the child to use to support them are being sought.

From the child's tinnitus booklet there will already be some information about how often the child is affected by tinnitus, times of day and places it occurs most often, and feelings associated with it. Visual images associated with it are also of great importance, whether negative or positive. If images are strong, then the use of visual imagery techniques is indicated in intervention. Through this process, it will have been discovered whether the child works best through play, drawing, visual imagery or a combination. The following case example is used to show how these can be used to change children's stories about tinnitus.

Case example: Scary monsters

Seven-year-old Hannah had a past history of intermittent conductive hearing loss and Eustachian tube dysfunction. She was troubled by intermittent tinnitus, which occurred both at school and at home. Hannah also described difficulties listening in the classroom, and keeping up with schoolwork. She was also distressed by her lack of friends, and was verbally teased at school. Both Hannah and her mother shared the belief that these difficulties had arisen as a result of her tinnitus. Hannah's teacher however, was surprised by her concerns, reporting that her schoolwork was average, but acknowledged Hannah's lack of friends.

Hannah was invited to play with a collection of soft toys. Talking as she played, it became clear that Hannah believed that the noises were the result of having a monster in her head. This was very scary for her, and was getting in the way of her concentration, listening, school work and friendships. Hannah selected a soft toy that she felt resembled her 'monster' and we seated this on the table in front of us. We used externalization techniques to think about the monster, what it was like, and to think of any times when the monster was not scary. We explained to Hannah what tinnitus was, and that there was not a real monster in her head; however, the noise at times might be so unpleasant that it seemed there was a monster there. Hannah was invited to talk to the monster, and to ask the monster to be her friend. Hannah gave the monster a name, and we were able to use the monster to fight the tinnitus noises. We thought about special powers that the monster might have, and how she might be able to get the monster to fight off the scary noises. This new story about the monster gave Hannah control over the scary noises.

For Hannah, the tinnitus noises were clearly frightening. Furthermore, both Hannah and her mother believed that tinnitus was the cause of her other difficulties. By changing tinnitus into something friendly and supportive, we were able to give Hannah a sense of power and influence over the tinnitus. Further sessions focused upon helping Hannah address the separate difficulties she had with friendships and school work.

Unique outcomes

During the process of assessment, the aim is to bring into the open the stories about tinnitus that are held by child and family. When tinnitus is troublesome, these stories will inevitably be problem-filled. We are listening out however, for examples of situations that contradict these dominant, problem-filled stories, and so bring to mind other, problem-free stories. For example, a child may hold a story that 'tinnitus always keeps them awake at night'. *Always?* If the child and family can think of a time when the child did get to sleep, even when the tinnitus was noisy, then we have begun to explore with them a new and different story from their dominating story that 'tinnitus stops you sleeping'. In narrative therapy these situations are called unique outcomes (White 1989). During intervention, as many and as varied unique outcomes as possible are explored in some depth, for each of the stories the child or family brings.

Mapping the influence of the 'problem' (tinnitus)

Tinnitus can have a significant effect upon a child's life, and its presence will inevitably affect the family also. No parent remains unaffected by seeing their child seemingly in pain, and distressed. Difficulties listening in school and getting to sleep at night are often mentioned as effects of tinnitus. Other difficulties in life, however, which may not be a direct outcome of tinnitus, can also become connected, or mapped onto the tinnitus. Tinnitus may have an impact that extends beyond the child experiencing the symptoms, and serve a function within the family which is unhelpful as the case example below shows.

Case example: Trouble at home

Ten-year-old Susie had tinnitus for as long as she could remember. Over the past year however, it had gradually worsened. Rarely present at school, it occurred most evenings at home. Susie's mother was worried about talking to her about the tinnitus for fear of making it worse. Instead, she would try to distract her by playing with her, or reading to her, often long into the night. Susie identified loud noises as triggering her tinnitus, and therefore the rest of the family were instructed to keep as quiet as possible. In particular, Susie identified arguments between Susie's father and her teenage brother as being the main influence upon her tinnitus. They frightened and worried her. Susie's brother however, was fed up with the limitations placed upon family life by Susie's tinnitus. As psychologists we can see that Susie's story about tinnitus was that it helped to prevent family arguments. For her brother, tinnitus was the source of their problems.

Externalizing

Narrative therapy holds the view that 'the person is never the problem; the problem is the problem' (White 1989). When a person sees a problem as an integral part of themselves, then it is difficult for them to change, or to believe that things can be different. It can be seen how tinnitus, by its very nature, can easily be viewed as an integral part of oneself, and hard to change.

Externalizing is the process of helping the person to separate from the problem, and to see the problem as something outside, and distinct from the person. This process of separation from the problem also helps relieve the person from all the negative thoughts, feelings and ideas about tinnitus with which they have become inextricably linked. White (1989) notes that externalizing helps to decrease conflict, and reduce feelings of failure, and stress. Thus, when working with children in this way, the tinnitus or problem is described in the third person; it is no longer ascribed to a person or relationship. In this way we do not say 'your tinnitus' but 'the tinnitus'. Care is taken not to use labels or diagnoses, as they internalize rather than externalize the problem. With younger children it is best to use the name that the child uses (e.g. one child named his tinnitus noises as 'boum boums'). By taking the problem outside of the person, it means that it can be influenced, and it does not add to a perception of helplessness.

Using externalizing as a technique for children allows the introduction of a more light-hearted and playful approach to therapy. The child can be invited to draw the tinnitus, so creating a depiction of the problem that can be looked at from outside the child. A toy can also be used to represent the tinnitus. The toy can be looked at and talked to, and new and different relationship can be explored with the tinnitus.

From our clinical experience, tinnitus symptoms often decrease when other presenting difficulties are also addressed alongside the therapy focusing on tinnitus (e.g. sleep, school difficulties, attention and listening skills, physical symptoms). For example, bullying is an issue for some children, with the bullies deliberately making loud noises to torment the child. Noise, absence of noise and stress are the most frequently cited factors associated with the onset of tinnitus episodes. These are often mentioned as precipitating the onset of tinnitus in schools, for example absence of background noise during tests or work periods, conversely high levels of noise in the playground, scraping noises or school bells. Helping teachers to understand each child's individual difficulties, often results in positive changes to classroom management.

Conclusions

Tinnitus is a common problem amongst hearing-impaired children and may cause sufficient distress or interference with everyday activities that intervention is required. Whilst traditional strategies may be effective for many children, there are some cases where additional psychological intervention is indicated. In this chapter we have presented a model of therapy for children with tinnitus that can be highly effective and produce a dramatic difference in the child's emotional or behavioural state within a few sessions. The focus is upon stories: the meanings, beliefs and emotions children, families and the wider network have about tinnitus. The aim is to bring to light the dominant stories that influence the child and family's response to tinnitus. Young children attempt to make sense of their tinnitus, and if adults fail to talk with them openly about tinnitus at the appropriate developmental level, the child will construct his or her own explanation. Tinnitus really can be a monster.

Although our clinical experience suggests that narrative therapy is effective in helping children cope with tinnitus, as we noted earlier, there is no empirical research base to support this. There is a great need for further research on all aspects of tinnitus in children, particularly in those with a hearing-impairment, including well-designed and conducted intervention studies.

8 Professional Issues

In the preceding chapters we have presented a number of psychological and clinical topics as they relate to deafness and deaf children. During the discussion of issues and suggestions for ways in which clinicians may work therapeutically with deaf children, we have assumed that readers may be experienced in working with deaf children but not in terms of their psychological or mental health needs, or conversely may be clinical, educational or counselling psychologists who are unfamiliar with working with deaf individuals. One of the aims of this book has been to provide some practical ideas of useful strategies and techniques to employ with deaf children, whilst being mindful of the fact that 'one size' does not fit all, and practitioners will need to be able to decide which strategies or techniques are appropriate for any individual case. There are a variety of therapeutic models or approaches (e.g. cognitive-behavioural therapy, narrative therapy, systemic therapy and individual psychodynamic psychotherapy) that may be of benefit to deaf children, some of which have been discussed at various points throughout this book, with consideration of how they might be adapted to accommodate the needs of deaf children. As yet there is no empirical evidence base on which to judge the relative efficacy of these differing approaches, so it is not possible to advocate the use of one over another. Indeed, the way in which therapists work is very much a matter of personal preference combined with training and the particular needs and orientation of the service. Further discussion of this issue will therefore have to wait until outcome studies are available for review.

The fact that a book such as this may be considered necessary is a reflection of the lack of formal training available in the field, and the paucity of suitably trained deaf practitioners. This leads to a number of dilemmas for professionals faced with a request to work with a deaf child and his or her family, when they may never have done so before. All psychologists, along with most other professions with responsibility for working with children, must adhere to their professional code of conduct and ethics which will have implications for their work with deaf children. However, they will also be working within a political context that influences the nature of services provided by health, education and social services. This will shape the nature of those services, to some extent determine the responsibilities of professionals, inform the expectations of service users and probably also impose restrictions on service delivery in some way. It is on these issues that this chapter will focus.

Political context

In the UK in recent years there have been a number of government reports, initiatives and policies pertaining to the health and welfare of children, that have particular implications for deaf children. The first, *Every Child Matters* (see http://www.everychildmatters.gov.uk), which was published in 2003, outlined the government's intention that every child should have the chance to reach his or her potential by reducing levels of educational failure and ill health. Recalling the research findings reviewed in Chapter 1 on the academic achievements of deaf children, and the significant proportion that have additional medical problems, it is clear that there is a way to go yet before these objectives are met. *Every Child Matters* states the need for an increase in child and adolescent mental health services (CAMHS) and improved speech and language therapy services, again both of which would be of immense value to deaf children and their families. The report also emphasizes the need for early identification of families in difficulty, and early intervention when needed. It recommends multi-disciplinary team-working, in locations convenient to families, such as schools, general practice surgeries or children's centres. It is hard to see how this latter goal can be achieved in the foreseeable future with the paucity of deaf health professionals and professionals trained to work therapeutically with deaf children and their families.

The next two major documents with particular relevance to deaf children form part of a series – the 'National Service Framework (NSF) for Children, Young People and Maternity Services' (2004). The most pertinent recommendations from *The Mental Health and Psychological Well-being of Children and Young People* document are summarized as follows:

- All staff should have the appropriate knowledge, training and experience to recognize early signs of deafness.

- Services should be flexible about where families are seen, for example at school, in the home or in family centres.

- Children with learning disabilities and mental health problems should have equal access to appropriate services, with effective coordination between these services.

- There should be a multi-agency approach to meeting need, that is, between health, education and social services, as required.

- Emphasis should be on preventative and early interventions.

- There should be sufficient appropriately trained staff.

This document also highlights the need for evidence-based practice and the importance of measuring outcomes of interventions from both the users' as well as service providers' perspectives. The report acknowledges the difficulties in achieving this, noting that children's problems often do not fit neatly into diagnostic categories, and that there is a high rate of co-morbidity of problems in children. This issue is particularly challenging in our work with deaf children, where outcome studies of therapeutic work are almost non-existent. The few exceptions to this have been noted elsewhere in this book (for example the PATHS® programme described in Chapter 2).

The other most relevant document in the NSF for Children series is entitled *Disabled Children and Young People and those with Complex Health Needs*. Irrespective of whether deafness is considered a disability, many deaf children do have multiple physical, medical, emotional and behavioural difficulties. In this document many of the recommendations mirror those in the previously cited one, in terms of early identification and intervention for families experiencing difficulties, locally provided services, appropriately trained staff and evidence-based care. Again, these goals are being achieved to a limited extent for many deaf children and their families at the present time. This document also points to the need for services for children with multiple needs to be well coordinated, high quality and family-centred and to promote social inclusion for all children. It states that commissioning of services for low incidence conditions (which arguably would include hearing-impairment, and certainly includes services such as cochlear implantation) should be coordinated on a regional or national basis to ensure equality of access to the services, and that the services are of equivalent quality. The importance of empowering families to make truly informed choices for their child is emphasized. The choices to be made by the parents of a deaf child are multiple and far-reaching, including whether to use sign language with their child, what type of education, and specific school they want for their child, whether to pursue cochlear implantation as an intervention, and so on. Over recent years, with the ever-increasing amount of information on the World Wide Web, the availability of information to enable parents to make informed choices has improved enormously. However, as always, it is often those families with the greatest needs who have the least access to information – those from ethnic minorities, those from lower socioeconomic backgrounds and the poorly educated.

Finally, this document also mentions the needs of siblings of children with complex needs. It acknowledges that they too may require support from child and adolescent mental health services. As we have seen previously, the siblings of deaf children may encounter a number of experiences that disadvantage them in some way, and a proportion may exhibit emotional or behavioural disturbance.

Although each of the documents mentioned above has relevance to deaf children, none of them is specifically aimed at this group. In contrast, the government document *Mental Health and Deafness: Towards Equity and Access: Best Practice Guidance* (Department of Health 2005) focuses solely on the needs of deaf people, but even so, is aimed primarily at those whose main mode of communication is BSL, and also pays relatively little attention to the specific needs of children (as opposed to adults). Having said this, it does call for better coordination of services (i.e. education, health, social services) when a child is identified as having a hearing-impairment, and informed choice for parents regarding decisions about, for example, education, echoing the edicts of the NSF. The *Towards Equity and Access* guidance advocates the need for deaf awareness training for all front-line health staff in primary and secondary care, for interpreters to be available for *all* health consultations and for more mental health workers to be trained in BSL. In addition, *Towards Equity and Access* states the need for greater emphasis on communication support in primary, secondary and further education, and later in employment, to prevent the social exclusion and isolation experienced by many deaf children and adults. We would wholeheartedly endorse this view, given the central role effective communication plays in all aspects of the deaf child's development and psychological well-being.

Training deaf clinical pyschologists

Approximately 50,000 deaf people in the UK use BSL as their first language (Health Advisory Service 1998). A significant proportion of deaf children (estimates of around 40%) will experience psychological or mental health problems at some point during their childhood. However, suitably qualified mental health professionals are a very rare commodity and there is currently only one dedicated mental health service for deaf children and their families, the National Deaf Service for Children. This multi-disciplinary service is based in London, although there are links between this service and two satellite ones in the North of England. There are obvious implications for accessibility for families needing these services, and undoubtedly a very great level of unmet need. Numbers of deaf social workers and teachers are comparatively high, with numbers of deaf counsellors also slowing increasing, but there are far fewer than needed to meet demand in their respective fields. At the present time in the UK there are less than a handful of qualified clinical psychologists who are deaf and use BSL as their primary means of communication.

The reasons for this extraordinarily small number are not clear but we can speculate that a number of factors are involved. First, the number of deaf people who have the necessary qualifications to apply for clinical psychology training courses is likely to be very small; the literacy achievements of many deaf young people preclude them from studying mainstream academic subjects at university, only a proportion will choose to study psychology and a smaller number still will want to train as clinical psychologists. However, this cannot be the whole story. Clinical psychology training courses have been obliged to give equal consideration to deaf applicants since the Disability Discrimination Act (1995), yet, until recently, deaf students appear to have applied for courses only very rarely. Atherton and Dent (2003) surveyed the 26 UK clinical psychology courses, of which 16 responded, regarding their experiences of interviewing and training deaf psychologists, using a combination of multi-choice and open-ended questions. They reported that although none of the courses used deafness as an exclusion criterion, only three courses had experience of interviewing a deaf applicant, and five courses said that they were 'unsure' whether they had ever had a deaf applicant. This study highlighted the variability with which courses provided deaf awareness training; half of the courses (eight) said that no training was given and a further two were 'unsure' whether it was or not.

A number of other issues have been highlighted by Atherton and Dent (2003) that may go some way towards explaining the rarity of deaf clinical psychologists. Although attitudes were generally positive towards training deaf clinical psychologists, the courses raised concerns about how a deaf trainee would communicate effectively with staff and other trainees during teaching sessions, largely due to the reliance on the spoken word. Poorly equipped teaching accommodation, in terms of specialist equipment (e.g. flashing fire alarms or loop systems), was also considered a potential problem. The use of sign language interpreting for teaching sessions was viewed with mixed feelings by the respondents.

The fundamental purpose of clinical psychology training is working therapeutically with a variety of clients – adults, children, the elderly and those with learning disabilities – in a variety of community and hospital settings. Experience is gained on a series of training 'placements'. Trainees typically complete five or six placements, where their work is supervised by a qualified clinical psychologist from the service, who discusses all aspects of the clinical and organizational work of the trainee in depth. Concerns were raised in the Atherton and Dent (2003) study regarding finding appropriate placements and supervisors, the impact an interpreter would have on the therapy process, and the trainee's ability to communicate effectively with a multi-disciplinary team. The issue of whether, once qualified, deaf clinical psychologists should, or would wish to, only work with deaf clients, was raised as a matter for discussion and debate.

Finally, in the current climate, at least in the UK, of restricted resources for all aspects of health care, the problem of acquiring the additional funding required to train a deaf clinical psychologist, for example to pay an interpreter, may play (an unacknowledged) role in the small numbers of trained deaf clinical psychologists.

This situation is likely to improve only very slowly, so in the meantime it is incumbent on those professionals with specialist knowledge and skills in working with deaf children and their families (whether deaf themselves or not) to support the training needs of deaf psychologists and other professionals potentially working therapeutically with deaf children, and to promote deaf awareness training as an essential part of training courses.

Roles, responsibilities and ethics

Professional ethics plays a role in the practice of psychological assessment and intervention with any client group, and although working with deaf children is not specifically the focus of ethical guidelines in the UK, ethical considerations are pertinent. Psychologists in the UK, USA and elsewhere are expected to adhere to codes of ethics and conduct set by their professional governing bodies (e.g. American Psychological Association 1992; British Psychological Society 2006b; National Association of School Psychologists 1992). Although differing in detail, in essence they are comparable.

It could be argued that one of the most fundamental standards relates to the psychologist's awareness of his or her own competencies, strengths and limitations arising from training, experience of differences in language or culture. Pertinent sections of the British Psychological Society's *Code of Ethics and Conduct* (2006b) standard of recognition of limits of competence (pp.15–16) states that psychologists should:

- practice within the boundaries of their competence

- remain abreast of scientific, ethical and legal innovations germane to their professional activities, with further sensitivity to ongoing

developments in the broader social, political and organizational
contexts in which they work

- seek consultation and supervision when indicated, particularly as
circumstances begin to challenge their scientific or professional
expertise

- engage in additional areas of professional activity only after
obtaining the knowledge, skill, training, education and experience
necessary for competent functioning

- remain aware of and acknowledge the limits of their methods, as
well as the limits of the conclusions that may be derived from such
methods under different circumstances and for different purposes.

In the UK, clinical psychology training does not include Deaf Studies as a man-
datory part of the course. Clinical psychologists therefore generally become
competent in working with deaf children or adults through 'on the job' experience and attendance at short courses, conferences and workshops relating to
deafness. A minority of psychologists may have completed a six-, or occasionally 12-month 'elective' training placement in a service for deaf children or
adults. In the USA, the competencies specific to working with deaf people are
given greater recognition than in the UK. The importance of communicative
competence is highlighted in the professional standards set for psychologists
working with hearing-impaired students, and specifically for school psychologists by the National Association of State Directors of Special Education
(NASDSE). They recommend that school psychologists be able to communicate
in the child's primary language or preferred mode of communication, be that
ASL, Total Communication (in its many forms), Sign Supported English (SSE),
or with whichever method the child is most comfortable. The NASDSE also
states that psychologists who provide services to deaf people should understand
the psychological, sociological, linguistic and cultural aspects of deafness, and
the implications of these factors. The communication policy of Gallaudet University (the world's only university for deaf students) School Psychology
Program goes further, with one of its recommendations being that it is the
ethical responsibility of school psychologists to recognize that despite training
and experience in the field, not all psychologists will have the communication
skills to work with every deaf, hard of hearing, or even hearing child, given the
diversity of communication methods used by children. Unlike in the UK, a few
specialized training programmes do exist in the USA for post-qualification
school psychologists and clinical psychologists. In the UK we have a way to go

yet in developing standards and training to meet the specific needs of deaf people.

One of the major roles of clinical psychologists working in any field, but especially those working with children, is psychological assessment. Assessment may take many forms (observation, interview, case history, use of standardized tests and questionnaires), serve a number of purposes (screening, diagnostic, evaluation of progress or intervention outcome or to inform intervention strategies), and may focus on one or more areas of functioning (behaviour, personality, academic achievement, intelligence or socio-emotional functioning). The conclusions drawn from these assessments often have implications that are far-reaching and may have a profound impact on the type and level of support, education or treatment a child receives. Therefore, it is essential that the assessment process is undertaken by professionals, including psychologists, with knowledge and understanding of the impact of hearing-impairment on the cognitive, behavioural, language and emotional development of children.

Particular issues arise when psychologists assess deaf children. We have discussed the caution with which results from norm-referenced tests should be administered and interpreted in Chapter 4, as very few of these tests provide norms for deaf children. If an interpreter has been used to assist in conducting an assessment, the nature of the interaction between the psychologist and the child is likely to have been altered. Seating arrangements that are necessary to accommodate the interpreter may make the demonstration of test items and presentation of test materials difficult. Using an interpreter for tests items that are timed may place the deaf child at a disadvantage, especially if instructions or information is provided part of the way through a task (e.g. 'You have one minute left'), as the child will have to look up to receive the information, and stop what they are working on, losing time. In terms of the translation itself, interpreting standardized test instructions into sign language will alter the message at a variety of levels, including syntactic, morphological and possibly semantic. In addition, the translation may inadvertently give the child clues or even the answer to the test item not conveyed by spoken instructions. For example, in a developmental assessment for very young children, the child may be asked to 'Show me your nose'. The interpreter may ask this question by signing 'Where your nose' – pointing to his or her nose!

Working with cultural and ethnic diversity

Throughout this book we have emphasized the importance of understanding and respecting the cultural, as opposed to the medical model, of deafness. All professionals working with deaf children and their families, including doctors, audiologists, psychologists, teachers, social workers and so on, should have received as a bare minimum, deaf awareness training and knowledge of the beliefs, values and attitudes of the Deaf community. However, clinicians working within the mental health field should arguably have a deeper level of understanding of the issues, and an awareness of the impact of living in the dominant hearing culture on deaf individuals. Glickman (1996, pp.115–153) states that:

> Culturally affirmative therapists strive to extend the relevancy and useful-ness of psychotherapy to culturally different people. They think about social structure, culture, power, and oppression and seek to intervene in ways that (a) are relevant and sensible to the client, (b) empower the clients and clients' community, (c) make connections between personal and collec-tive experience, and (d) balance cultural and clinical considerations.

Sue and Sue (2003, p.18) state that in order to be a competent mental health professional working with members of a different culture to one's own, the practitioner must be aware of his or her own assumptions, values and biases in relation to the other culture. This can be an uncomfortable process, but one that can be discussed within supervision sessions. They (p.16) also discuss the pre-requisites for successful therapeutic interventions with families with deaf members, using a multi-cultural therapeutic approach they define as 'both a helping role and process that uses modalities and defines goals consistent with the life experiences and cultural values of clients, recognizes client identities to include individual, group and universal dimensions'. They suggest that it is essential that the therapist understands and can share the worldview of his or her clients. This does not mean that therapists should necessarily hold this worldview; rather they must accept these views in a non-judgemental manner. Therapeutic effectiveness will be enhanced if the therapist is able to agree inter-vention goals and treatment strategies that are consistent with the cultural values of the client. For example, in terms of a deaf child, the goal of an intervention may be to improve the child's communication skills within lessons at school. If this child has culturally Deaf parent(s), this may mean advocating provision of appropriate sign language input at school rather than speech and language therapy sessions to improve speech intelligibility.

For some deaf children, belonging to the Deaf culture is not the only minority group with whom they must assimilate. In the UK, USA and elsewhere, there is diversity in racial, ethnic and religious backgrounds amongst deaf/Deaf individuals. Children growing up in families that are part of two minority cultures are at risk of experiencing double discrimination and disadvantage. Some deaf children and their families face discrimination by members of their own ethnic group due to beliefs held by the ethnic community about dis-ability or deafness. Thus, deaf children from ethnic minorities may experience oppression, marginalization and racism from a variety of sources, including the Deaf community itself.

Access to mental health services by families from ethnic minorities is typically more difficult than for families from the majority (usually white) culture. Not surprisingly, deaf ethnic minority children are even less likely to receive the mental health care they need. Clinicians with expertise in working with children in these circumstances are a rarity indeed. It is unrealistic if not unreasonable to expect mental health workers to become experts in every possible cultural background and therefore at times it may be necessary to seek the advice of an 'elder' of the community, whilst being mindful of issues of confidentiality.

In terms of the development of a cultural identity in minority groups faced with oppression by a dominant culture, Sue and Sue (2003, p.214) propose a five-stage concept framework designed to help therapists understand their client's culture-based attitudes and behaviours. The five stages are (1) conformity, (2) dissonance, (3) resistance and immersion, (4) introspection and (5) integrative awareness. In the first stage, members of a cultural minority have a preference for the cultural values of the dominant culture over those of their own culture, and may hold negative views of their own culture (or that of their parents). In the dissonance stage the individual is exposed to views, attitudes and beliefs of the minority culture that conflict with those of the dominant culture leading to questioning and challenging of those views. The next stage is characterized by feelings of guilt, shame and anger as the individual recognizes that their previously held beliefs and attitudes devalue their cultural heritage. This results in a swing to unquestioning endorsement of the minority culture values and strong anti-dominant culture feelings. In the final two stages the individual begins to question group views and becomes selective about those they wish to endorse, eventually understanding and valuing aspects of both their own and the dominant culture.

This is clearly a sophisticated model of identity development that is potentially helpful in understanding the development of a strong Deaf identity, and is most likely to be pertinent when working with adolescents and young adults, rather than children. However, therapists working with younger deaf children should be mindful of the impact the child's experiences within their family, educational environment and wider community may be having on their identity development in the longer term. Also, therapists working with deaf children from immigrant or ethnic minority cultures may find it helpful to consider these stages when trying to understand and formulate the problems presented by these children. Therapists should also reflect on their own stage of cultural identity development as a member of the majority or dominant culture (if indeed they are), and consider whether this has implications for their ability to work effectively with a particular child or family.

Working with interpreters

Having argued the case for the need for sufficient numbers of mental health professionals to be trained to work with deaf children and their families, it must be acknowledged that given current resources, it is likely that many interventions will be undertaken by non-specialists in deafness and practitioners who cannot communicate fluently in BSL. For some deaf children, for example those for whom sign language is a second language learnt later in childhood or used only to supplement spoken English, therapists with a moderate level of skill in BSL may be able to communicate effectively with the child. However, if there is any possibility that the therapist's skills are less advanced than the child's, a qualified BSL interpreter must be used. This is obviously also the case if any other family member, or individual attending appointments, communicates primarily/most comfortably in BSL. It is not adequate to assume that the deaf child or adult is able to lip-read, as even those who are proficient at lip-reading will miss a considerable proportion of what is said. It is also not good practice to rely solely on written communication – first, this slows communication down to such an extent that engagement and rapport are likely to be compromised, and second, the literacy skills of some deaf individuals are inadequate for this method to convey the subtleties typically required in psychological interventions. Occasional use of written communication may be appropriate to clarify or check understanding.

Although an obvious and pragmatic solution to the need for an interpreter may be to use the child's classroom sign interpreter, a member of their family, or a family friend, this is not appropriate. The child may find it difficult to talk freely in front of these people, or have fears about confidentiality that will impact on treatment effectiveness. Also the adults have a dual relationship with the child and may have difficulty remaining neutral as a result of emotional involvement with the child. In addition, when employing a sign language interpreter it is important to be mindful of the fact that the Deaf community is a small one, and the deaf child or his or her parents may know the interpreter in a non-professional capacity, again potentially leading to concerns regarding confidentiality or impartiality, despite the code of ethics interpreters must adhere to.

Professional interpreters are trained to a very high level for comprehension and accuracy. When working in the medical or mental health fields it is desirable for them to have additional training in medical and psychiatric/psychological terminology and issues. Interpreters also need particular skills in working with children whose use of language may be very idiosyncratic or inconsistent. They need to be able to take into account the child's age and developmental level, vocabulary and educational level. Flexibility is essential as the child may use home signs or incorrectly formed signs that the interpreter will need to work out the meaning of, and explain to other participants in the session. The interpreter can thus provide the therapist with useful insights into the child's language and communication abilities.

Within therapy sessions, the presence of an interpreter may have an impact on the therapeutic process. In early sessions the child may develop greater rapport and trust with the interpreter than with the therapist, as this is with whom they are primarily communicating. If the intervention is with the whole family, that is, family or systemic therapy, the therapist may need to reflect on this with the family as part of the intervention. As the National Child Traumatic Stress Network White Paper (NCTSN 2006) notes, the interpreter may become the object of transference or experience counter-transference (the unconscious redirection of the child's feelings for a significant person in their lives onto the therapist, and the redirection of the therapist's feelings onto the child or family member respectively). In other words, the interpreter may trigger a strong emotional response, either positive or negative, from the child or other family member. Equally, the interpreter may experience uncomfortable or unhelpful feelings towards the child or family member. The therapist will need to identify and address these issues within the sessions, or if more appropriate, with the interpreter after the session. In any case, it is important to allow sufficient time after sessions to debrief the interpreter, especially if the session has contained distressing material.

Consultative/liaison model of intervention

As we have seen, a serious shortage of professionals trained to work with deaf children and their families with mental health or psychological difficulties exists in the UK and elsewhere. When a specialist in the field is not available to work with the child directly, a consultation or liaison model of intervention can often be successfully employed. Clinicians with experience and expertise in deafness, along with child development, learning difficulties or child mental health can provide advice, supervision and support to a range of professionals with training in mental health but no specialist knowledge of deafness and its impact on development. Professionals involved in a consultation model of intervention could include school teachers and counsellors, educational psychologists and members of a child and adolescent mental health service multi-disciplinary team – clinical psychologists, social workers, psychiatrists, nurses, family therapists and other therapists.

Consultation may be provided on a variety of levels, from advice on deaf awareness and optimizing communication, to in-depth supervision of an ongoing therapeutic intervention or assessment. Specific issues on which consultation may be provided include the implications of language deficits and communication difficulties on socio-emotional development and learning. This is of pertinence to all professional groups who may work with deaf children only rarely, as they are unlikely to have received training in this area on generic courses (e.g. mainstream classroom teachers or nurses). Understanding of this area is vital as it underpins so much of the rest of the work with deaf children. The advice of psychologists who are experienced in assessing deaf children should be sought by colleagues who do not have this expertise, particularly over issues such as the choice of appropriate psychometric assessments for a specific child. Advice regarding adaptation of the tests where necessary, the interpretation of test results and even report writing can be provided. Another area where psychologists unused to working with deaf children may not feel confident is in diagnosing an autism spectrum disorder in a deaf child. Although we have sought to provide information on issues such as these in this book, we do not advocate a 'cookbook approach' to assessing a deaf child and the procedures we have outlined are intended as general guidance rather than prescriptive instructions.

Consultation between professionals (of any combination) can occur through a variety of mechanisms. The most common and straightforward is probably the case conference where the professionals involved with the child, possibly along with the child's parents, meet on a number of occasions to discuss the needs of the child and plan and monitor a programme of assessment and/or intervention. Second, experienced professionals in the field of deafness may jointly run clinics with professionals at a local level, for example in child and adolescent mental health service clinics or general practice surgeries or family centres. If such clinics occur on a sufficiently regular basis with a stable group of personnel, knowledge and skills can be transferred so that the consultant support can gradually be reduced. Finally, a recent development in the UK has been to provide a telemedicine service using video-conferencing technology for deaf children experiencing psychological difficulties, in a defined geographical area in the north of England, through links to the National Deaf Service for Children based in London. Where necessary, individual therapy for deaf children with mental health problems can be provided by the London clinicians using the video link. Unfortunately the service is currently considered a pilot and is being evaluated in order to ascertain whether continued funding is warranted.

There are a number of benefits to the consultation model of intervention. The increased knowledge and understanding of Deaf culture by local non-specialist professionals is likely to have a positive impact on their ability to empathize and engage with deaf individuals, improving the therapeutic alliance. Working closely with experienced therapists can lead to increased motivation and confidence, which is in turn likely to lead to greater satisfaction in working with deaf children and their families. Frustrations and feelings of helplessness or being de-skilled are more likely to be avoided if inexperienced therapists are given appropriate support and advice. In addition, providing services to deaf children at a local level, rather than by specialist services may be experienced as less stigmatizing and result in easier access to the service for the family – more frequent appointments and fewer difficulties attending them.

Whilst these benefits may be appealing, there are also a number of potential problems to consider. If there is no standard process or mechanism by which consultation services are provided or funded this could lead to inequalities of access for families living in different areas of the country. Clarity is needed over who pays for the service, along with adequate time for the clinicians to provide the service if their role is not one dedicated to providing a consultation service. In many instances consultation is currently provided by clinicians to profession-als employed by organizations/hospitals other than their own, and therefore consultation work is in addition to their contracted work. These are issues that need to be resolved at a national rather than a local level to ensure that services for deaf children are provided in a way that is equitable, accessible and of consis-tently high quality for all children in need of them.

Conclusions

Hearing-impaired children are likely to be disadvantaged in many ways from birth onwards: their hearing loss may not be identified in a timely fashion (despite Universal Newborn Hearing Screening Programmes), they may not have access to good communication or language models when in their infant and pre-school years, they may have other physical disabilities or medical problems, or may have no deaf peers with whom they can identify. In turn, dis-advantages such as these are likely to have an impact on the child's development – socially, emotionally, psychologically and behaviourally. As a result, a signifi-cant proportion of hearing-impaired children develop educational, psychologi-cal or mental health problems requiring input from a variety of professionals and services. Sadly, and most unfairly, these children are further disadvantaged by the lack of accessible services available to meet their needs in these areas. Although commissioners of services recognize the need for professionals with appropriate training and experience to provide services to deaf children, the reality is that many deaf children have needs that cannot currently be met by the few specialist services that exist in the UK. The result is that hearing-impaired children and their families may need to be seen and helped through a variety of non-specialist services, in a range or settings and by professionals with diverse backgrounds and training. This can be a very positive and effective process, providing that information, advice and support is available to those clinicians who need it, including easy, reliable access to interpreters when necessary. The diversity and complexity of psychological work with hearing-impaired children and their families is daunting at times, and certainly stimulating and challenging, even for practitioners with considerable experience in the field. However, the potential for making a positive contribution to the lives of deaf children and their families is great, and well worth investment in training and resources.

References

Achenbach, T.M. (1991a) *Integrative Guide for the 1991 CBCL/4–18, YSR and TRF Profiles.* Burlington, VT: University of Vermont Department of Psychiatry.

Achenbach, T.M. (1991b) *Manual for the Youth Self-report and 1991 Profile.* Burlington, VT: University of Vermont Department of Psychiatry.

Achenbach, T.M. (1992) *Manual for the Child Behaviour Checklist/2–3 and 1992 Profile.* Burlington, VT: University of Vermont Department of Psychiatry.

Adams, W. and Sheslow, D. (1995) *Wide Range Assessment of Visual-Motor Abilities.* London: Harcourt Assessment.

ADPS (2006) *National Surrey.* Available at: www.education.ed.ac.uk/adps/survey/index.shtml, accessed on 19 November 2007.

Ainsworth, M.D.S. and Bell, S.M. (1970) 'Attachment, exploration and separation: illustrated by the behaviour of one-year-olds in a strange situation.' *Child Development 41,* 49–67.

Aksoy, S., Akdogan, O., Gedikli, Y. and Belgin, E. (2007) 'The extent and levels of tinnitus in children of central Ankara.' *International Journal of Pediatric Otorhinolaryngology 71,* 263–268.

American Psychiatric Association (1994) *Diagnostic and Statistical Manual of Mental Disorders, Fourth Edition*™. Washington, DC: American Psychiatric Association.

American Psychological Association (1992) *Ethical Principles of Psychologists and Code of Conduct.* Washington, DC: APA.

American Speech-Language-Hearing Association (2005) *(Central) Auditory Processing Disorders – The Role of the Audiologist* [Position statement]. Available at: www.asha.org/docs/html/PS2005-00114.html, accessed on 19 November 2007.

Antia, S.D. and Kriemeyer, K.H. (2003) 'Peer interactions of deaf and hard-of-hearing children.' In M. Marschark and P.E. Spencer (eds) *Oxford Handbook of Deaf Studies, Language, and Education.* Oxford: Oxford University Press.

Aplin, D.Y. (1987) 'Classification of dyspraxia in hearing-impaired children using the Q-technique of factor analysis.' *Journal of Child Psychology and Psychiatry 28,* 581–596.

Atherton, R. and Dent, A. (2003) 'Training deaf clinical psychologists.' *Clinical Psychology 32,* 17–20.

Aust, G. (2002) 'Tinnitus in childhood.' *International Tinnitus Journal 8,* 20–26.

Badian, N.A. (1984) 'Reading disability in an epidemiological context: incidence and environmental correlates.' *Journal of Learning Disabilities 17,* 129–136.

Bailey, A., Le Couteur, A., Gottesman, I., Bolton, P., *et al.* (1995) 'Autism as a strongly genetic disorder: evidence from a British twin study.' *Psychological Medicine 25,* 63–77.

Ballantine, J. (1981) 'Acceptance of deafness in deaf adolescents: a repertory grid study.' *South African Journal of Communication Disorders 28,* 53–58.

Baron-Cohen, S. (2003) *Mind Reading: An Interactive Guide to Emotion.* London: Jessica Kingsley Publishers.

Baron-Cohen, S. and Swettenham, J. (1996) 'The relationship between SAM and ToMM: two hypotheses.' In P. Carruthers and P.K. Smith (eds) *Theories of Theories of Mind.* Cambridge: Cambridge University Press.

Bat-Chava, Y. (1993) 'Antecedents of self-esteem in deaf people: a meta-analytic review.' *Rehabilitation Psychology 38*, 221–234.

Bayer, J.K., Hiscock, H., Hampton, A. and Wake, M. (2007) 'Sleep problems in young infants and maternal mental and physical health.' *Journal of Paediatrics and Child Health 43*, 66–73.

Bayley, N. (2005) *Bayley Scales of Infant and Toddler Development.* Third Edition. Oxford: Harcourt Assessment.

Beazley, S. and Moore, M.M. (1995) *Deaf Children, Their Families and Professionals: Dismantling Barriers.* London: Fulton Publishers.

Beck, J.S., Beck, A.T., Jolly, J. and Steer, R. (2005) *Beck Youth Inventories – Second Edition for Children and Adolescents.* Oxford: Harcourt Assessment.

Beitchman, J.H. (1985) 'Therapeutic considerations with the language impaired preschool child.' *Canadian Journal of Psychiatry 30*, 546–553.

Bellman, M., Lingham, S. and Aukett, A. (1996) *Schedule of Growing Skills II.* London: nferNelson.

Berg, I.K. and Steiner, T. (2003) *Children's Solutions Work.* New York: WW Norton & Co. Ltd.

Bishop, D.V.M. (1983) 'Comprehension of English syntax by profoundly deaf children.' *Journal of Child Psychology and Psychiatry 24*, 415–434.

Bolea, A.S., Felker, D.W. and Barnes, M. (1971) 'A pictorial self-concept scale for children in K-4.' *Journal of Educational Measurement 8*, 223–224.

Briscoe, J., Bishop, D.V. and Norbury, C.F. (2001) 'Phonological processing, language, and literacy: a comparison of children with mild-to-moderate sensorineural hearing loss and those with specific language impairment.' *Journal of Child Psychology and Psychiatry 42*, 329–340.

British Psychological Society (2006a) *Autistic Spectrum Disorders: Guidance for Chartered Psychologists Working with Children and Young People.* BPS Position Paper. London: British Psychological Society.

British Psychological Society (2006b) *Code of Ethics and Conduct.* London: British Psychological Society.

Broesterhuizen, M.L. (1997) 'Psychological assessment of deaf children.' *Scandinavian Journal of Audiology Suppl. 46*, 43–49.

Bruininks, R. and Bruininks, B. (2005) *Bruininks-Oseretsky Test of Motor Proficiency.* Second Edition. London: nferNelson.

Buhrmann, V. (1979) 'Early recognition of infantile autism.' *South African Medical Journal 56*, 18, 724–727.

Carpenter, M., Nagell, K. and Tomasello, M. (1998) 'Social cognition, joint attention, and communicative competence from 9 to 15 months of age.' *Monographs of the Society for Research in Child Development 63*.

Cates, J. (1991) 'Self-concept in hearing and pre-lingual, profoundly deaf students.' *American Annals of the Deaf 136*, 352–359.

Chakrabarti, S. and Fombonne, E. (2005) 'Pervasive developmental disorders in preschool children: confirmation of high prevalence.' *American Journal of Psychiatry 162*, 1133–1141.

Chamberlain, C., Morford, J.P. and Mayberry, R.I. (eds) (2000) *Language Acquisition by Eye.* Mahwah, NJ: Lawrence Erlbaum Associates.

Chermak, G.D. (2001) 'Auditory processing disorder: an overview for the clinician.' *The Hearing Journal 54*, 11–22.

Chermak, G.D. and Musiek, F.E. (1997) *Central Auditory Processing Disorders: New Perspectives.* San Diego, CA: Singular Publishing Group.

Coggins, T.E. and Carpenter, R.L. (1981) 'The communicative intention inventory: a system for observing and coding children's early intentional communication.' *Applied Psycholinguistics 2*, 182–197.

Cohen, N.J. (1996) 'Unsuspected language impairments in psychiatrically disturbed children: developmental issues and associated conditions.' In J.H Beitchman, N.J. Cohen, M.M. Konstantareas and R. Tannock (eds) *Language, Learning and Behavior Disorders: Developmental, Biological and Clinical Perspectives.* Cambridge: Cambridge University Press.

Conners, C.K. (1997) *Conners' Rating Scales – Revised.* New York: Multi-Health Systems Inc.

Connor, C.M., Craig, H.K., Raudenbush, S.W., Heavner, K. and Zwolan, T.A. (2006) 'The age at which young deaf children receive cochlear implants and their vocabulary and speech-production growth: is there an added value for early implantation?' *Ear and Hearing 27,* 628–644.

Coopersmith, S. and Gilberts, R. (1982) *Behavioural Academic Self-esteem: A Rating Scale* (manual). Palo Alto, CA: Consulting Psychologists Press.

Cope, N., Harold, D., Hill, G., Moskvina, V., *et al.* (2005) 'Strong evidence that KIAA0319 on chromosome 6p is a susceptibility gene for developmental dyslexia.' *American Journal of Human Genetics 76,* 581–591.

Courtin, C. and Melot, A.M. (2005) 'Metacognitive development of deaf children: lessons from the appearance-reality and false-belief task.' *Developmental Science 8,* 16–25.

Craig, H. (1965) 'A sociometric investigation of the self-concept of the deaf child.' *American Annals of the Deaf 110,* 456–470.

Crowe, T.V. (2003) 'Self-esteem scores among deaf college students: an examination of gender and parents' hearing status and signing ability.' *Journal of Deaf Studies and Deaf Education 8,* 199–206.

Davis, J.M., Elfenbein, J.L., Chum, R.S. and Bentler, R. (1986) 'Effects of mild and moderate hearing impairments on language, educational, and psychosocial behaviour of children.' *Journal of Speech and Hearing Disorders 51,* 53–62.

Davis, L.J. (2007) 'Deafness and the riddle of identity.' *The Chronicle of Higher Education.* Available at: http://chronicle.com/weekly/V53/i19/19b00601.htm, accessed on 11 July 2007.

Department of Health (2003) *Every Child Matters.* London: DoH.

Department of Health (2004) *National Service Framework for Children, Young People and Maternity Services.* Autism Exemplar (Sept. 2004). London: DoH.

Department of Health (2005) *Mental Health and Deafness: Towards Equity and Access.* London: DoH.

Desselle, D.D. (1994) 'Self-esteem, family climate, and communication patterns in relation to deafness.' *American Annals of the Deaf 139,* 322–328.

Diggle, T., McConachie, H.R. and Randle, V.R.L. (2007) 'Parent-mediated early intervention for young children with autism spectrum disorder.' *Cochrane Database of Systematic Reviews 2,* Art. No: CD003496. DOI: 10.1002/14651858.CD003496.

Disability Discrimination Act (1995) London: The Stationery Office.

Dodd, B., Hua, Z., Crosbie, S., Holm, A. and Ozanne, A. (2002) *Diagnostic Evaluation of Articulation and Phonology.* Oxford: Harcourt Assessment.

Drukier, G. (1989) 'The prevalence and characteristics of tinnitus with profound sensorineural hearing impairment.' *American Annals of the Deaf 134,* 260–264.

Dyck, M.J. and Denver, E. (2003) 'Can the emotion recognition ability of deaf children be enhanced? A pilot study.' *Journal of Deaf Studies and Deaf Education 8,* 348–356.

Dyck, M.J., Farrugia, C., Shochet, I.M. and Holmes-Brown, M. (2004) 'Emotion recognition/understanding ability in hearing or vision-impaired children: do sounds, sights or words make the difference?' *Journal of Child Psychology and Psychiatry 45,* 789–800.

Dyspraxia Foundation (n.d.) 'What is Dyspraxia?' Available at: www.dyspraxiafoundation.org.uk/services/dys_dyspraxia.php, accessed on 21 November 2007.

Easterbrooks, S.R. and Stephenson, B. (2006) 'An examination of twenty literacy, science and mathematics practices used to educate students who are deaf or hard of hearing.' *American Annals of the Deaf 151,* 385–397.

Eder, R.A. (1990) 'Uncovering young children's psychological selves: individual and developmental differences.' *Child Development 61,* 849–863.

Edwards, L.C. (2004) 'Neuropsychological development of hearing-impaired children.' In S. Austen and S. Crocker (eds) *Deafness in Mind: Working Psychologically with Deaf People Across the Lifespan.* London: Whurr Publishers.

Edwards, L.C. (2007) 'Children with cochlear implants and complex needs: a review of outcome research and psychological practice.' *Journal of Deaf Studies and Deaf Education 12,* 258–268.

Edwards, L., Frost, R. and Witham, F. (2006) 'Developmental delay and outcomes in paediatric cochlear implantation: implications for candidacy.' *International Journal of Pediatric Otorhinolaryngology 70,* 1593–1600.

Edwards, S., Fletcher, P., Garman, M., Hughes, A., Letts, C. and Sinka, I. (1997) *Reynell Developmental Language Scales III.* London: nferNelson.

Elliot, C.D., Smith, P. and McCulloch, K. (1996) *British Ability Scales: Second Edition.* London: nferNelson.

Erikson, E. (1968) *Identity: Youth and Crisis.* New York: Norton.

Evans, J.W. (1989) 'Thoughts on the psychosocial implications of cochlear implantation in children.' In E. Owens and D.K. Kessler (eds) *Cochlear Implants in Young Deaf Children.* Boston: College-Hill, pp.307–314.

Fombonne, E. (2005) 'Epidemiology of autistic disorder and other pervasive developmental disorders.' *Journal of Clinical Psychiatry 66,* Suppl. 10, 3–8.

Fombonne, E., Zakarian, R., Bennett, A., Meng, L. and McLean-Heywood, D. (2006) 'Pervasive developmental disorders in Montreal, Quebec, Canada: prevalence and links with immunizations.' *Pediatrics 118,* e139–150.

Fortnum, H. and Davis, A. (1997) 'Epidemiology of permanent childhood hearing impairment in Trent Region, 1985–1993.' *British Journal of Audiology 31,* 409–446. Erratum in: *British Journal of Audiology* (February 1998) *32,* 1, 63.

Fortnum, H.M., Marshall, D.H. and Summerfield, A.Q. (2002) 'Epidemiology of the UK population of hearing-impaired children, including characteristics of those with and without cochlear implants – audiology, aetiology, comorbidity and affluence.' *International Journal of Audiology 41,* 170–179.

Francks, C., Paracchini, S., Smith, S.D., Richardson, A.J., *et al.* (2004) 'A 77-kilobase region of chromosome 6p22.2 is associated with dyslexia in families from the United Kingdom and the United States.' *American Journal of Human Genetics 75,* 1046–1058.

Fransella, F., Bell, R. and Banister, D. (2004) *A Manual for Repertory Grid Technique.* Chichester: John Wiley and Sons.

Frederickson, N., Frith, U. and Reason, R. (1999) *Phonological Assessment Battery.* London: nferNelson.

Freeman, R.D., Malkin, S.F. and Hastings, J.O. (1975) 'Psychosocial problems of deaf children and their families: a comparative study.' *American Annals of the Deaf 120,* 275–304.

Fujiki, M., Brinton, B., Morgan, M. and Hart, C.H. (1999) 'Withdrawn sociable behaviour of children with language disorder.' *Language Speech and Hearing Services in Schools 30,* 183–195.

Fundudis, T., Kolvin, I. and Garside, R. (1979) *Speech Retarded and Deaf Children: Their Psychological Development.* London: Academic Press.

Gallaudet Research Institute (2005) *Regional and National Summary Report of Data from the 2004–2005 Annual Survey of Deaf and Hard of Hearing Children and Youth.* Washington, DC: GRI, Gallaudet University.

Garcia, R. and Turk, J. (2007) 'The applicability of Webster-Stratton Parenting Programmes to deaf children with emotional and behavioural problems, and autism, and their families: annotation and case report of a child with autistic spectrum disorder.' *Clinical Child Psychology and Psychiatry 12,* 125–136.

Geers, A.E. (2006) 'Factors influencing spoken language outcomes in children following early cochlear implantation.' *Advances in Otorhinolaryngology 64,* 50–65.

Geers, A. and Moog, J. (1989) 'Factors predictive of the development of literacy in profoundly hearing-impaired adolescents.' *The Volta Review 91,* 69–86.

Giallo, R. and Gavidia-Payne, S. (2006) 'Child, parent and family factors as predictors of adjustment for siblings of children with a disability.' *Journal of Intellectual Disability Research 50*, 937–948.

Gibbs, S. (2004) 'The skills in reading shown by young children with permanent and moderate hearing impairment.' *Educational Research 46*, 17–24.

Gioia, G.A., Isquith, K., Guy, S.C. and Kenworthy L. (2000) *Behaviour Rating Inventory of Executive Function.* London: Harcourt Assessment.

Glickman, N.S. (1996) 'The development of culturally affirmative Deaf identities.' In N.S. Glickman and M.A. Harvey (eds) *Culturally Affirmative Psychotherapy with Deaf Persons.* Mahwah, NJ: Erlbaum.

Glickman, N. and Carey, J. (1993) 'Measuring Deaf cultural identities: a preliminary investigation.' *Rehabilitation Psychology 38*, 275–283.

Glover, D.M. (2003) 'The deaf child – challenges in management: a parent's perspective.' *International Journal of Pediatric Otorhinolaryngology 67S1*, S197–S200.

Goodman, R. (1997) 'The Strengths and Difficulties Questionnaire: a research note.' *Journal of Child Psychology and Psychiatry 38*, 581–586.

Graham, J.M. (1987) 'Tinnitus in hearing impaired children.' In J. Hazell (ed.) *Tinnitus.* London: Churchill Livingstone.

Graham, J. (2004) 'Medical and physiological aspects of deafness.' In S. Austen and S. Crocker (eds) *Deafness in Mind: Working Psychologically with Deaf People Across the Lifespan.* London: Whurr Publishers.

Graham, J. and Butler, J. (1984) 'Tinnitus in children.' *Journal of Laryngology and Otology. Supplement 9*, 236–241.

Greenberg, M.T. (1978) 'Attachment behaviour, communicative competence, and parental attitudes in preschool deaf children.' Dissertation, University of Virginia.

Greenberg, P. and Kusche, C. (1998) 'Preventive intervention for school-age deaf children: the PATHS curriculum.' *Journal of Deaf Studies and Deaf Education 3*, 49–63.

Griffiths, R. (1984) *Griffiths Mental Development Scales. The Abilities of Young Children.* Oxford: The Test Agency.

Grigorenko, E.L., Wood, F.B., Golovyan, L., Meyer, M., Romano, C. and Pauls, D. (2003) 'Continuing the search for dyslexia genes on 6p.' *American Journal of Medical Genetics. Part B Neuropsychiatric Genetics 118*, 89–98.

Hadadian, A. (1995) 'Attitudes towards deafness and security of attachment relationships among young deaf children and their parents.' *Early Education and Development 6*, 181–191.

Hallam, R.S. (1987) 'Psychological approaches to the evaluation and management of tinnitus distress.' In J. Hazell (ed.) *Tinnitus.* London: Churchill Livingstone.

Happé, F. (1994) 'Advanced test of theory of mind: understanding of story characters' thoughts and feelings by able autistic, mentally handicapped and normal children and adults.' *Journal of Autistic and Developmental Disorders 24*, 129–154.

Happé, F. (1995) 'The role of age and verbal ability in theory of mind task performance of subjects with autism.' *Child Development 66*, 843–855.

Harter, S. (1986) 'Processes underlying the construction, maintenance, and enrichment of the self-concept in children.' In J. Suls and A. Greenwald (eds) *Psychological Perspectives on the Self,* Vol. 3. London: Lawrence Erlbaum.

Hatcher, P.J., Hulme, C., Miles, J.N.V., Carroll, J.M., *et al.* (2006) 'Efficacy of small group reading intervention for beginning readers with reading-delay: a randomized controlled trial.' *Journal of Child Psychology and Psychiatry 47*, 820–827.

Haynes, C. and Naidoo, S. (1991) 'Children with specific speech and language impairment.' *Clinics in Developmental Medicine No 119.* Oxford: MacKeith Press/Blackwell Scientific.

Health Advisory Service (1998) *Forging New Channels: Commissioning and Delivering Mental Health Services for People who are Deaf.* London: British Society for Mental Health and Deafness.

Hellman, S.A., Chute, P.M., Kretschmer, R.E., Nevins, M.E., Parisier, S.C. and Thurston, L.C. (1991) 'The development of a Children's Implant Profile.' *American Annals of the Deaf 136*, 77–81.

Henderson, S.E. and Sugden, D. (1992) *Movement Assessment Battery for Children.* London: Harcourt Assessment.

Heyman, I., Fombonne, E., Simmons, H., Ford, T., Meltzer, H. and Goodman, R. (2001) 'Prevalence of obsessive-compulsive disorder in the British nationwide survey of child mental health.' *British Journal of Psychiatry 179*, 324–329.

Hindley, P. (1997) 'Psychiatric aspects of hearing-impairments.' *Journal of Child Psychology and Psychiatry 38*, 101–117.

Hindley, P.A. and Kroll, L. (1998) 'Theoretical and epidemiological aspects of attention deficit and overactivity in deaf children.' *Journal of Deaf Studies and Deaf Education 3*, 64–72.

Hindley, P.A., Hill, P.D., McGuigan, S. and Kitson, N. (1994) 'Psychiatric disorder in deaf and hearing children and young people: a prevalence study.' *Journal of Child Psychology and Psychiatry 35*, 917–934.

Hiscock, H., Canterford, L., Ukoumunne, O.C. and Wake, H. (2007) 'Adverse associations of sleep problems in Australian preschoolers: national population study.' *Pediatrics 119*, 86–93.

Holgers, K.-M. (2003) 'Tinnitus in 7-year-old children.' *European Journal of Pediatrics 162*, 276–278.

Holgers, K.-M. and Juul, J. (2006) 'The suffering of tinnitus in childhood and adolescence.' *International Journal of Audiology 45*, 267–272.

Holgers, K.-M., Erlandsson, S.I. and Barrenas, M.L. (2000) 'Predictive factors for the severity of tinnitus.' *Audiology 39*, 284–291.

Hume [1748] (1999) *An Enquiry Concerning Human Understanding: Oxford Philosophical Texts.* Ed. T.L Beauchamp. Oxford: Oxford University Press.

International Dyslexia Association (2002) Just the Facts: Definition of Dyslexia. Available at: www.interdys.org/ewebeditpro5/upload/Definition_of_Dyslexia.pdf, accessed on 21 November 2007.

Israelite, N., Ower, J. and Goldstein, G. (2002) 'Hard-of-hearing adolescents and identity construction: influences of school experiences, peers and teachers.' *Journal of Deaf Studies and Deaf Education 7*, 134–148.

Jackson, A.L. (2001) 'Language facility and theory of mind development in deaf children.' *Journal of Deaf Studies and Deaf Education 6*, 161–176.

Jambor, E. and Elliott, M. (2005) 'Self-esteem and coping strategies among deaf students.' *Journal of Deaf Studies and Deaf Education 10*, 63–81.

Jansson-Verkasalo, E., Ceponiene, R., Valkama, M., Vainionpaa, L., *et al.* (2003) 'Deficient speech-sound processing, as shown by the electrophysiologic brain mismatch negativity response, and naming ability in prematurely born children.' *Neuroscience Letters 4*, 5–8.

Jastreboff, P.J. (1990) 'Phantom auditory perception (tinnitus): mechanisms of generation and perception.' *Neuroscience Research 8*, 221–254.

Jerger, J. and Musiek, F. (2000) 'Report of the consensus conference on the diagnosis of auditory processing disorders in school-aged children.' *Journal of the American Academy of Audiology 11*, 467–474.

Jocelyn, L.J., Casiro, O.G., Beattie, D., Bow, J. and Kneisz, J. (1998) 'Treatment of children with autism: a randomised controlled trial to evaluate a caregiver-based intervention program in community day-care centers.' *Journal of Developmental and Behavioral Pediatrics 19*, 326–334.

Jure, R., Rapin, I. and Tuchman, R.F. (1991) 'Hearing impaired autistic children.' *Developmental Medicine and Child Neurology 33*, 1062–1072.

Katz, J., Stecker, N.A. and Henderson, D. (1992) 'Introduction to central auditory processing.' In J. Katz, N.A. Stecker and D. Henderson (eds) *Central Auditory Processing: A Transdisciplinary View.* St Louis, MO: Mosby Year Book, Inc.

Kelly, D.P., Kelly, B.J., Jones, M.L., Moulton, N.J., Verhulst, S.J. and Bell, S.A. (1993) 'Attention deficits in children and adolescents with hearing loss. A survey.' *American Journal of Diseases of Children 147*, 737–741.

Kelly, G.A. (1955) *The Psychology of Personal Constructs.* New York: W.W. Norton.

Kentish, R. and Crocker, S.R. (2005) 'Scary monsters and waterfalls: tinnitus narrative therapy for children.' In R. Tyler (ed.) *Tinnitus Treatment.* New York: Thieme.

Kentish, R., Crocker, S. and McKenna, L. (2000) 'Children's experience of tinnitus: a preliminary survey of children presenting to a psychology department.' *British Journal of Audiology 34*, 335–340.

Khan, S., Edwards, L. and Langdon, D. (2005) 'The cognition and behaviour of children with cochlear implants, children with hearing aids and their hearing peers: a comparison.' *Audiology and Neuro-otology 10*, 117–126.

Knutson, J.F., Johnson, C.R. and Sullivan, P.M. (2004) 'Disciplinary choices of mothers of deaf children and mothers of normally hearing children.' *Child Abuse and Neglect 28*, 925–937.

Korkman, M., Kirk, U. and Kemp, S. (1998) *NEPSY: A Developmental Neurological Assessment. The Psychological Corporation.* Oxford: Harcourt Assessment.

Kurtzer-White, E. and Luterman, D. (2003) 'Families and children with hearing loss: grief and coping.' *Mental Retardation and Developmental Disabilities Research Reviews 9*, 232–235.

Ladd, P. (2002) *Understanding Deaf Culture: In Search of Deafhood.* Cleveden: Multilingual Matters Ltd.

Lane, H. (1990) 'Cultural and infirmity models of deaf Americans.' *Journal of the Academy of Rehabilitative Audiology 23*, 11–26.

Lederberg, A.R. and Everhart, V.S. (1998) 'Communication between deaf children and their hearing mothers: the role of language, gesture, and vocalizations.' *Journal of Speech, Language and Hearing Research 41*, 887–899.

Linder, T.W. (1993) *Transdisciplinary Play-based Assessment. A Functional Approach to Working with Young Children.* Baltimore, MD: Paul H. Brookes Publishing Co.

Lord, C., Rutter, M. and LeCouteur, A. (1994) 'Autism Diagnostic Interview – Revised.' *Journal of Autism and Developmental Disorders 24*, 659–686.

Lord, C., Risi, S., Lambrecht, L., Cook, E.H. Jr., *et al.* (2000) 'The Autism Diagnostic Observation Schedule-Generic: a standard measure of social and communication deficits associated with the spectrum of autism.' *Journal of Autism and Developmental Disorders 30*, 205–223.

Lowe, M. and Costello, A.J. (1995) *Symbolic Play Test: Second Edition.* London: nferNelson.

Marcia, J.E. (1993) *The Relational Roots of Identity.* London: Lawrence Erlbaum Associates.

Marschark, M. (2003) 'Cognitive functioning in deaf adults and children.' In M. Marschark and P.E. Spencer (eds) *Oxford Handbook of Deaf Studies, Language, and Education.* Oxford: Oxford University Press.

Marschark, M., Green, V., Hindmarsh, G. and Walker, S. (2000) 'Understanding theory of mind in children who are deaf.' *Journal of Child Psychology and Psychiatry 41*, 1067–1073.

Martin, D. and Bat-Chava, Y. (2003) 'Negotiating deaf–hearing friendships: coping strategies of deaf boys and girls in mainstream schools.' *Child: Care, Health and Development 29*, 511–521.

Martin, K. and Snashall, S. (1994) 'Children presenting with tinnitus: a retrospective study.' *British Journal of Audiology 28*, 111–115.

Martinez Devesa, P., Waddell, A., Perera, R. and Theodoulou, M. (2007) 'Cognitive behavioural therapy for tinnitus.' *Cochrane Database of Systematic Reviews, Issue 1.* Art. No.: CD005233. DOI: 10.1002/14651858.CD005233.pub2.

Mayberry, R.I. (2002) 'Cognitive development in deaf children: the interface of language and perception in neuropsychology.' In S.J. Segalowitz and I. Raplin (eds) *Handbook of Neuropsychology Second Edition, Vol. 8, Part II.* Amsterdam: Elsevier Science.

McConkey Robbins, A., Koch, D.B., Osberger, M.J., Zimmerman-Phillips, S. and Kishon-Rabin, L. (2004) 'Effect of age at cochlear implantation on auditory skill development in infants and toddlers.' *Archives of Otolaryngology, Head and Neck Surgery 130*, 570–574.

McPhillips, M., Hepper, P.G. and Mulhern, G. (2000) 'Effects of replicating primary-reflex movements on specific reading difficulties in children: a randomized, double-blind controlled trial.' *The Lancet 355*, 537–541.

Medical Research Council Institute of Hearing (2004) *APD Booklet.* Available at: www.ihr.mrc.ac.uk/research/projects/apd/documents/APD_Booklet.pdf, accessed on 22 November 2007.

Miller, N. (1986) *Dyspraxia and its Management.* London: Croom Helm.

Mills, R.P., Albert, D.M. and Brain, C.E. (1986) 'Tinnitus in childhood.' *Journal of Clinical Otolaryngology 11*, 431–434.

Mills, R.P. and Cherry, J.R. (1984) 'Subjective tinnitus in children with otological disorders.' *International Journal of Pediatric Otorhinolaryngology 7*, 21–27.

Mitchell, R.E. and Karchmer, M.A. (2002) 'Chasing the mythical ten percent: parental hearing status of deaf and hard of hearing students in the United States'. Available at: http://gri.gallaudet.edu/Demographics/SLS_Paper.pdf, accessed on 10 July 2007.

Moeller, M.P. and Schick, B. (2006) 'Relations between maternal input and theory of mind understanding in deaf children.' *Child Development 77*, 751–766.

Mundy, P., Sigman, M. and Kasari, C. (1994) 'Joint attention, developmental level, and symptom presentation in autism.' *Development and Psychopathology 6*, 394–401.

Musselman, C., MacKay, S., Trehub, S.C. and Eagle, R.S. (1996) 'Communicative competence and psychosocial development in deaf children and adolescents.' In J.H. Beitchman, N.J. Cohen, M.M. Konstantareas and R. Tannock (eds) *Language, Learning and Behavior Disorders: Developmental, Biological and Clinical Perspectives.* Cambridge: Cambridge University Press.

National Association of School Psychologists (1992) *Professional Conduct Manual.* Silver Spring, MA: NASP Publications.

National Initiative for Autism: Screening and Assessment (2003) *National Autism Plan for Children.* London: National Autistic Society.

NCTSN (2006) *Addressing the Trauma Treatment Needs of Children who are Deaf or Hard of Hearing and the Hearing Children of Deaf Parents. Revised.* Los Angeles, CA, and Durham, NC: National Child Traumatic Stress Network.

NDCS (2003a) *Parenting and Deaf Children: A Psychosocial Literature-based Framework.* London: National Deaf Children's Society.

NDCS (2003b) *Parenting and Deaf Children: Report of the Needs Assessment Study Undertaken as Part of the NDCS Parents' Toolkit Development Project.* London: National Deaf Children's Society.

Neale, M.D. (1997) *Neale Analysis of Reading Ability.* Second Edition. London: nferNelson.

Newman, P.R. and Newman, B.M. (1976) 'Early adolescence and its conflict: group identity versus alienation.' *Adolescence 11*, 261–274.

NHS Executive (1996) *Clinical Guidelines: Using Clinical Guidelines to Improve Patient Care Within the NHS.* London: NHS Executive.

Nikolaraizi, M. and Hadjikakou, K. (2006) 'The role of educational experiences in the development of deaf identity.' *Journal of Deaf Studies and Deaf Education 11*, 477–492.

NIMHE/DH (2005) *Towards Equity and Access, Best Practice Guidelines.* London: National Institute for Mental Health in England and Department of Health.

Nodar, R.H. and Lezak, M.H.W. (1984) 'Paediatric tinnitus: a thesis revised.' *Journal of Laryngology and Otology, Supplement 9*, 234–235.

O'Connor, P.D., Sofo, F., Kendall, L. and Olsen, G. (1990) 'Reading disabilities and the effects of colored filters.' *Journal of Learning Disabilities 23*, 597–603.

Pennington, B.F. (1991) *Diagnosing Learning Disorders.* New York, NY: Guilford Press.

Peterson, C.C. (2002) 'Drawing insight from pictures: the development of concepts of false belief in children with deafness, normal hearing, and autism.' *Child Development 73*, 5, 1442–1459.

Peterson, C.C. (2004) 'Theory of mind development in oral deaf children with cochlear implants or conventional hearing aids.' *Journal of Child Psychology and Psychiatry 45*, 1096–1106.

Peterson, C.C. and Siegal, M. (1995) 'Deafness, conversation and theory of mind.' *Journal of Child Psychology and Psychiatry 36*, 3, 459–474.

Peterson, C.C. and Siegal, M. (2000) 'Insights into a theory of mind from deafness and autism.' *Mind and Language 15*, 123–145.

Peterson, C.C., Wellman, H.M. and Liu, D. (2005) 'Steps in theory-of-mind development for children with deafness or autism.' *Child Development 76*, 502–517.

Piers, E. (1984) *Manual for the Piers-Harris Children's Self-concept Scale.* Los Angeles, CA: Western Psychological Services.

Pipp-Siegel, S. (2000) 'Resolution of grief of parents with young children with hearing loss.' Unpublished manuscript. Boulder, CO: University of Colorado.

Powell, J.E., Edwards, A., Edwards, M., Pandit, B.S., Sungum-Palwal, S.R. and Whitehouse, W. (2000) 'Changes in the incidence of childhood autism and other autistic spectrum disorders in preschool children from two areas of the West Midlands.' *Developmental Medicine and Child Neurology 42*, 624–628.

Pressman, L., Pipp-Siegel, S., Yoshinaga-Itano, C., Kubicek, L. and Emde, R.N. (2000) 'A comparison of links between emotional availability and language gain in young children with and without hearing loss.' *The Volta Review 100*, 251–278.

Prezbindowski, A.K., Adamson, L.B. and Lederberg, A.R. (1998) 'Joint attention in deaf and hearing 22-month-old children and their hearing mothers.' *Journal of Applied Developmental Psychology 19*, 377–387.

Prizant, B.M. and Schuler, A. (1997) 'Facilitating communication: language approaches.' In D.J. Cohen and A.M. Donnellan (eds) *Handbook of Autism and Developmental Disorders.* New York: John Wiley and Sons.

Reynell, J. (1979) *Manual for the Reynell-Zinkin Scales for Young Visually Handicapped Children.* Windsor: NFER.

Richardson, A.J. (2004) 'Clinical trials of fatty acid treatment in ADHD, dyslexia, dyspraxia and the autistic spectrum.' *Prostaglandins, Leukotrienes and Essential Fatty Acids 70*, 383–390.

Risch, N., Spiker, D., Lotspeich, L., Nouri, N., *et al.* (1999) 'A genomic screen of autism: evidence for a multilocus etiology.' *American Journal of Human Genetics 65*, 493–507.

Roid, G.H. and Miller, L.J. (1997) *Examiner's Manual, Leiter International Performance Scale – Revised.* Wheat Lane, IL: Stoelting Company.

Rosenberg, M. (1965) *Society and the Adolescent Self-Image.* Princeton, NJ: Princeton University Press.

Russell, P.A., Hosie, J.A., Gray, C.D., Hunter, N. *et al.* (1998) 'The development of theory of mind in deaf children.' *Journal of Child Psychology and Psychiatry 39*, 903–910.

Rutter, M. (2005) 'Aetiology of autism: findings and questions.' *Journal of Intellectual Disability Research 49*, 231–238.

Rutter, M. and Mawhood, L. (1991) 'The long-term sequelae of specific developmental disorders of speech and language.' In M. Rutter and P. Casaer (eds) *Biological Risk Factors in Childhood and Psychopathology.* Cambridge: Cambridge University Press.

Sackett, D.L., Rosenberg, W.M.C., Gray, J.A.M., Haynes, R.B. and Richardson, W.S. (1996) 'Evidence-based medicine: what it is and what it isn't.' *British Medical Journal 312*, 71–72.

Sackett, D.L., Straus, S.E., Richardson, W.S., Rosenberg, W. and Haynes, R.B. (2000) *Evidence-based Medicine: How to Practice and Teach EBM. Second Edition.* Edinburgh: Churchill Livingstone.

Sahli, S. and Belgin, E. (2006) 'Comparison of self-esteem level of adolescents with cochlear implant and normal hearing.' *International Journal of Pediatric Otorhinolaryngology 70*, 1601–1608.

Sanchez, L. and Stephens, D. (1997) 'A tinnitus problem questionnaire in a clinic population.' *Ear and Hearing 18*, 210–217.

Savastano, M. (2007) 'Characteristics of tinnitus in childhood.' *European Journal of Pediatrics 166*, 8, August.

Semel, E., Wiig, E.H. and Secord, W. (2006) *Clinical Evaluation of Language Fundamentals*. Fourth UK Edition. Oxford: Harcourt Assessment.

Sharma, M., Purdy, S.C., Newall, P., Wheldall, K., Beaman, R. and Dillon, H. (2006) 'Electrophysiological and behavioural evidence of auditory processing deficits in children with reading disorder.' *Clinical Electrophysiology 117*, 1130–1144.

Shin, M.S., Kim, S.K., Kim, S.S., Park, M.H., Kim, C.S. and Oh, S.H. (2007) 'Comparison of cognitive function in deaf children between before and after cochlear implant.' *Ear and Hearing 28* (Suppl.) 22S–28S.

Shulman, C., Bukai, O. and Tidhar, S. (2007) 'Communicative intent in autism.' In E. Schopler, N. Yirmiya, C. Shulman and L.M. Marcus (eds) *The Research Basis for Autism Intervention*. New York: Kluwer Academic/Plenum Publishers.

Silvestre, N., Ramspott, A. and Pareto, I.D. (2006) 'Conversational skills in a semistructured interview and self-concept in deaf students.' *Journal of Deaf Studies and Deaf Education 12*, 38–54.

Smith, T., Groen, A.D. and Wynn, J.W. (2000) 'Randomized trial of intensive early intervention for children with pervasive developmental disorder.' *American Journal of Mental Retardation 105*, 269–285.

Snijders, J.T., Tellegen, P.J. and Laros, J.A. (1989) *Snijders-Oomen Non-verbal Intelligence Test: SON-R 5½–17. Manual and Research Report*. Groningen: Wolters-Noordhoff.

Snowling, M., Slothard, S. and McLean, J. (1996) *Graded Non-word Reading Test*. London: Harcourt Assessment.

Spangler, T.H. (1987) 'Exploration of the relationship between deaf children's attachment classification in the strange situation and effects of parents' success in grieving and coping.' Dissertation, Los Angeles, CA.

Spencer, P.E. (2000) 'Looking without listening: is audition a prerequisite for normal development of visual attention during infancy?' *Journal of Deaf Studies and Deaf Education 5*, 291–302.

Stallard, P. (2002) *Think Good – Feel Good: A Cognitive Behaviour Therapy Workbook for Children and Young People*. Chichester: John Wiley & Sons Ltd.

Sterne, A. and Goswami, U. (2000) 'Phonological awareness of syllables, rhymes, and phonemes in deaf children.' *Journal of Child Psychology and Psychiatry 41*, 609–625.

Stevenson, J. (1996) 'Developmental changes in the mechanisms linking language disabilities and behaviour disorders.' In J.H. Beitchman, N.J. Cohen, M.M. Konstantareas and R. Tannock (eds) *Language, Learning and Behavior Disorders: Developmental, Biological and Clinical Perspectives*. Cambridge: Cambridge University Press.

Stevenson, J. and Richman, N. (1978) 'Behaviour, language and development in three-year-old children.' *Journal of Autism and Childhood Schizophrenia 8*, 299–313.

Stoneman, Z. (2005) 'Siblings of children with disabilities: research themes.' *Mental Retardation 43*, 339–350.

Stouffer, J.L., Tyler, R.S., Booth, J.C. and Buckrell, B. (1992) 'Tinnitus in normal-hearing and hearing-impaired children'. In J.M. Aran and R. Dauman (eds) *Proceedings of the Fourth International Tinnitus Seminar*. The Netherlands: Kugler & Ghedini Publications, 255–258.

Sue, D.W. and Sue, D. (2003) *Counseling the Culturally Diverse: Theory and Practice, Fourth Edition*. New York: J. Wiley and Sons.

Surowiecki, V.N., Sarant, J., Maruff, P., Blamey, P.J., Busby, P.A. and Clark, G.M. (2002) 'Cognitive processing in children using cochlear implants: the relationship between visual memory, attention, and executive functions and developing language skills.' *Annals of Otology, Rhinology and Laryngology Supplement 189*, 119–126.

Sween, E. (1999) 'The one-minute question: What is narrative therapy? Some working answers.' In D. Denborough and C. White (eds) *Extending Narrative Therapy: A Collection of Practice Based Papers*. Adelaide: Dulwich Centre Publications.

Tellegen, P.J., Winkel, M., Wijnberg-Williams, B. and Laros, J.A. (1998) *Snijders-Oomen Non-verbal Intelligence Test: SON–R 2½–7. Manual and Research Report*. Lisse: Swets and Zeitlinger.

Thoutenhoofd, E. (2006) 'Cochlear implanted pupils in Scottish schools: 4-year school attainment data (2000–2004).' *Journal of Deaf Studies and Deaf Education 11*, 171–188.

Thoutenhoofd, E.D., Archbold, S.M., Gregory, S., Lutman, M.E., Nikolopoulos, T.P. and Sach, T.H. (2005) *Paediatric Cochlear Implantation: Evaluating Outcomes*. London: Whurr Publishers.

Torgesen, J.K., Wagner, R. and Rashotte, C. (1999) *Test of Word Reading Efficiency*. London: Harcourt Assessment.

Transler, C., Gombert, J.E. and Leybaert, J. (2001) 'Phonological decoding in severely and profoundly deaf children: similarity judgment between written pseudowords.' *Applied Psycholinguistics 22*, 61–82.

Tyler, R.S. and Baker, L.J. (1983) 'Difficulties experienced by tinnitus sufferers.' *Journal of Speech and Language Research 8*, 150–154.

Vacarri, C. and Marschark, M. (1997) 'Communication between parents and deaf children: implications for social-emotional development.' *Journal of Child Psychology and Psychiatry 38*, 793–801.

van Gurp, S. (2001) 'Self-concept of deaf secondary school students in different educational settings.' *Journal of Deaf Studies and Deaf Education 6*, 54–69.

van Uden, A. (1983) *Diagnostic Testing of Deaf Children. The Syndrome of Dyspraxia*. Lisse: Swets and Zeitlinger.

Vostanis, P., Hayes, M., Du Feu, M. and Warren, J. (1997) 'Detection of behavioural and emotional problems in deaf children and adolescents: comparison of two rating scales.' *Child: Care, Health and Development 23*, 233–246.

Vygotsky, L. (1986) *Thought and Language*. Cambridge, MA: MIT Press.

Wagner, R., Torgesen, J. and Rashotte, C. (1999) *Comprehensive Test of Phonological Processing*. London: Harcourt Assessment.

Wallis, D., Musselman, C. and MacKay, S. (2004) 'Hearing mothers and their deaf children: the relationship between early, ongoing mode match and subsequent mental health functioning in adolescents.' *Journal of Deaf Studies and Deaf Education 9*, 2–14.

Way, N. and Robinson, M.G. (2003) 'A longitudinal study of the effects of family, friends, and school experiences on the psychological adjustment of ethnic minority, low SES adolescents.' *Journal of Adolescent Research 18*, 324–346.

Webster, A. (1994) 'Hearing impairment.' In J. Solity and G. Bickler (eds) *Support Services: Issues for Health and Social Services Professionals*. London: Cassell.

Webster-Stratton, C. (1984) 'Randomized control trial of two-parent-training programs for families with conduct-disordered children.' *Journal of Consulting and Clinical Psychology 52*, 666–678.

Wechsler, D. (1993) *Wechsler Objective Reading Dimensions*. Oxford: Harcourt Assessment.

Wechsler, D. (2004) *Wechsler Intelligence Scale for Children*. Fourth UK Edition. Oxford: Harcourt Assessment.

Wechsler, D. (2005) *Wechsler Individual Achievement Test*. Oxford: Harcourt Assessment.

Wetherby, A., Cain, D.H., Yonclas, D.G. and Walker, V.G. (1988) 'Analysis of intentional communication of normal children from the prelinguistic to the multiword stage.' *Journal of Speech and Hearing Research 31*, 240–252.

White, D., Leach, C., Sims, R., Atkinson, M. and Cottrell, D. (1999) 'Validation of the Hospital Anxiety and Depression Scale for use with adolescents.' *British Journal of Psychiatry 175*, 452–454.

White, M. (1989) 'The externalizing of the problem and the re-authoring of lives and relationships.' In M. White *Selected Papers*. Adelaide: Dulwich Centre Publications.

Williams, D.P., Williams, A.R., Graff, J.C., Hanson, S., *et al.* (2002) 'Interrelationships among variables affecting well siblings and mothers in families of children with a chronic illness or disability.' *Journal of Behavioural Medicine 25*, 411–424.

Woodward, K. (1997) 'Concepts of identity and difference.' In K. Woodward (ed.) *Identity and Difference*. Thousand Oaks, CA: Sage.

Woolfe, T. (2001) 'The self-esteem and cohesion to family members of deaf children in relation to the hearing status of their parents and siblings.' *Deafness and Education International 3*, 80–95.

Woolfe, T., Want, S.C. and Siegal, M. (2002) 'Signposts to development: theory of mind in deaf children.' *Child Development 73*, 768–778.

World Health Organization (1992) *The ICD-10 Classification of Mental and Behavioural Disorders*. Geneva: World Health Organization.

Yirmiya, N., Erel, O., Shaked, M. and Solomonica-Levi, D. (1998) 'Meta-analyses comparing theory of mind abilities of individuals with autism, individuals with mental retardation, and normally-developing individuals.' *Psychological Bulletin 124*, 283–307.

Yoshinaga-Itano, C. (2001) 'The social-emotional ramifications of universal newborn hearing screening, early identification and intervention of children who are deaf or hard of hearing.' *A Sound Foundation Through Early Amplification – Proceedings of the Second International Conference*. pp.221–231. Available at: www.audiologyonline.com/articles/pf_article_detail.asp?article_id=1305, accessed on 10 July 2007.

Zigmond, A.S. and Snaith, R.P. (1983) 'The Hospital Anxiety and Depression Scale.' *Acta Psychiatrica Scandinavica 67*, 452–454.

Subject Index

Author Index